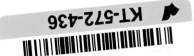

Teaching Motor Skills to Children with Cerebral Palsy

and Similar Movement Disorders

Teaching Motor Skills to Children with Cerebral Palsy

and Similar Movement Disorders

A Guide for Parents and Professionals

Sieglinde Martin

Woodbine House   2006

All rights reserved under International and Pan American Copyright Conventions. Published in the United States by Woodbine House, Inc., 6510 Bells Mill Rd., Bethesda, MD 20817. 800-843-7323. www.woodbinehouse.com

Library of Congress Cataloging-in-Publication Data

Martin, Sieglinde.
  Teaching motor skills to children with cerebral palsy and similar movement disorders : a guide for parents and professionals / Sieglinde Martin.— 1st ed.
      p. cm.
  Includes bibliographical references and index.
  ISBN-13: 978-1-890627-72-0
  ISBN-10: 1-890627-72-0
  1. Cerebral palsied children—Rehabilitation. 2. Cerebral palsy—Exercise therapy. 3. Movement disorders in children—Patients—Rehabilitation. 4. Movement disorders in children—Exercise therapy. 5. Physical therapy for children. 6. Physical therapy for infants. I. Title.
  RJ496.C4M293 2006
  618.92'836—dc22

                                                                                2006007196

Printed in the United States of America

First edition

10 9 8 7 6 5 4 3 2

This book is dedicated to the wellbeing and happiness of children with cerebral palsy.

Table
of
Contents

Preface and Acknowledgements

"I wish there were a book that explains to parents what we do and why we do it," I complained. "You just have to write it, " Michelle Byars retorted. "Yes, you write it," Mike Jewell chimed in. "If you write another book I want to be part of it," Lisa Barnett added. That was the casual workplace exchange among therapists that took place almost three years ago.

Doing two things at once—tuning into the child I was treating and explaining to the parent what I was doing and why it was important for the home program to be done in a similar way—had never been easy for me. Even now, as a senior therapist, it remained a frustrating challenge for me. A clear, practical, easy-to-read book on the subject would help everyone—physical therapists, parents, and their children with cerebral palsy and similar movement disorders, as well as other professionals working with the children. And so the work started.

Having help from colleagues was wonderful. I wanted to speak for as many of us as possible and not just present my own perspective and experience. Having dedicated therapists like Lisa, Michelle, and Cherri Willsey read and reread, critique, edit, and approve the first chapters was very valuable. I thank them and also Christie Johnson, Anne Cain-Sheban, Kim Hamilton-Holmes, Jennie Jacobs, and Linda Lowes Pax for reading all or part of the book and providing their input. Jennie's many practical suggestions and Linda's sharp checking-the-facts scrutiny were welcome and helpful. Marilyn Wikoff provided help concerning wheelchair exercises and transfers. My daughter, Kristine Martin, helped with the initial patient summaries. I am grateful to Lisa Barnett for contributing Chapter 17, which provides information about current medical management and bracing.

Even with so many therapists helping, much more had to be done. I thank Susan Harryman, the seasoned pediatric physical therapist from the Kennedy Krieger Institute in Baltimore, who peer-reviewed and edited the manuscript. Susan worked patiently with me during the summer months of 2005. Susan's and my total of 60 years of experience in the field came to consensus on matters small and large. I am thankful to Nancy Gray Paul, the acquisition editor from Woodbine House, for her good foresight in having someone like Susan assist me.

Next, illustrations were needed for the many home exercises. I thank Harcourt Assessment, Inc., for allowing me to use photos for my book, *Pediatric Balance Program,* which had not been published, in it. Tanya Corzatt, a professional photographer, did most of these photos, and her son Camdon was the patient model. I also thank Allison Fuchs, and the parents of Joseph Sheridan, Katie Lackey, Chelsea Swallow, Samantha Stando, Jordan Moore, Kaily Boutinot, and Mary Kate Bunstine for allowing me to use their photos.

These photos were good to have, but many more were needed. I am indebted to my colleagues at Columbus Children's Hospital and in the School system for providing many valuable contacts to families they worked with.

I thank all of the parents who opened their homes and were willing to demonstrate exercises. Their enthusiasm and support for my project made the many photo trips in Spring and Summer of 2005 a wonderful experience, which I will cherish all my life. For their warm welcome, I thank Carrie and Rob Beyer and their son Sam; Augustine Bonsy and her son Jeffrey; Maria D'Amore and her daughter Marina; Rachael Estepp and her son Wyatt; Amy Frick and her daughter Alexandra; Marietta Harper and her grandson Reese Harper; Peg Hart and her son Benjamin; Melissa Herbert and her son Joe; Jennifer Kemp and her son Andrew; Suzanne Ruschau and her daughter Sophia; Sandhya Jakkam and her son Rajshekhar; Linda Searles and her son Matthew; Brenda and Terry Winebrenner and their son Caleb; and Carrie Whitman and her daughter Brenna.

I tried not to impose for more than an hour on these wonderful parents' busy schedules. For some families this meant several visits. My special thanks to Michelle Fenstermaker and her son Jack for modeling exercises and sharing family photos, and to Lynne Fogel and her daughter Erica for lasting through two tedious range of motion photo sessions with good cheer. More special thanks to Michael and Laura Henderson and their son Bryce; Chris and Mike Miller and their daughter Grace; Crystal Thompson and her son Chase; and Tanya and Rob Corzatt and their son Camdon for showing me their creative home activity adaptations which came to enrich the book. I thank my daughter Heide Martin for doing some of the home visit photography.

At times, drawings were needed for a clear presentation. I thank P. Jason Sauer and Mary Newman for creating fine illustrations.

My helpful colleagues, my friend Mirjam Gerber, and my dear husband, Gerhard Martin, offered helpful language corrections, for which I am thankful. But would a person without any background in medicine or rehabilitation find the text easy to read? Wren Grigore of Venice, Florida, tackled this issue with enthusiasm and energy. With her good sense of language and organization, Wren did invaluable editing work as I was trying to get chapters ready for Woodbine House. Susan Stokes, my compassionate editor from Woodbine House, continued and completed the editing work. Being a mother of a child with special needs, she looked at the text from a parent's point of view—asking probing questions, clearing up possible points of misunderstandings, adding words for parents, and reorganizing chapters and exercises as needed. Thank you.

For the appealing layout and cover design, I thank Brenda Ruby from Woodbine House.

This book is done, but the work to improve the skill of children with cerebral palsy is not. Readers and users of this book are encouraged to send feedback to *sieglindemartin@sbcglobal.net.*

Sieglinde Martin, June 2006

Introduction

Amber was born almost three months premature. Too young to breathe on her own, she spent her first five weeks in an incubator. Amber's parents spent many anxious hours at the hospital. There were complications, but Amber survived. Her parents were happy to take her home at last. With their good care, Amber started to thrive. She gained weight, grew, and developed into a cute, alert baby.

Now seven months old, Amber loves to be held and carried. When her mother is busy in the kitchen, Amber likes to be in her infant seat close by and watch her. She also likes to sit in her baby swing and listen to music. Amber is a happy baby but her parents have started to worry again. During Amber's last doctor's visit the physician had placed her on her tummy. When Amber only briefly lifted her head, he told them that her development seemed to be delayed and referred her for a physical therapy evaluation. What would the physical therapist do? Make Amber stronger? They think Amber is pretty strong already. When they stand her up, she strongly straightens her back and legs and holds herself up.

Amber's parents have made the appointment as suggested, but are skeptical about it.

Luke is two and a half years old and big for his age. But he does not yet walk. To get around, he crawls or walks with a walker. Still, his parents are glad he has this much mobility. There was a time he did much less.

Luke had been born on time, weighing a healthy 7 lbs. He had spent less than a day at the hospital before he and his mother were brought home by his happy father. But fate was cruel. Two weeks later the family was in a car accident with serious consequences. Luke sustained a head injury. A subdural bleed, a subarachnoid bleed, and cerebral edema were diagnosed. Luke spent ten days in the hospital. Afterwards, a physical therapist began *coming to the house—first once a month, and then two times a week after an evaluation showed that Luke's motor development was not progressing as it should.*

Now the therapist comes to their house three times a week, and, as before, the visits are paid for by their state's Medicaid system. Luke's parents feel lucky but still have complaints. At times the physical therapy visits interfere with their family plans. Also the therapist keeps telling them things to do with Luke. They like to help Luke, but would rather do it on their own terms. Luke really likes his physical therapy visits and looks forward to them, but his parents feel the therapist is playing with him too much and does not have him work as he should. With all the therapy, they wonder, why isn't he walking?

Derek is already five years old and goes to kindergarten. But he still is the baby of the family. Everyone loves Derek and dotes over him. When Derek needs something, his sisters rush to get it. His dad still carries him when they go out. At dinnertime his mom helps him to climb into his seat. There is a reason for this. Derek has cerebral palsy. Born after a hard labor, he developed slower than his sisters had. His legs in particular had always felt stiff.

When Derek was not crawling and sitting by nine months of age, his parents became concerned and the pediatrician referred him for a pediatric physical and occupational therapy evaluation. Ever since, his parents have taken him to weekly physical therapy and occupational therapy sessions. For two years Derek also had speech therapy. The therapies have helped Derek. They also have been very valuable to his parents. They helped them understand Derek's problems as well as how to help him learn all the things he needed to learn.

Now, Derek is walking short distances without support. His parents no longer take him to the clinic for therapy. Instead, he receives occupational and physical therapy at school. What a relief not to have to drag him to all his appointments any more! Derek goes to afternoon kindergarten. In the morning after his sisters have left for school, Derek is free to play with his toys, and his mother is free to read the paper or call a friend. After years of hectic schedules, she enjoys this freedom. But then again she feels unsure. "Is this good for Derek? Shouldn't I do more for him?" she wonders. She misses the weekly contact with Derek's therapists and the guidance they gave her. She does not yet know Derek's school physical therapist well and finds it difficult to contact her.

If you have a child like Amber, Luke, or Derek, you probably can relate to the stories above. Perhaps you have been informed that your child has a developmental delay, cerebral palsy, or another condition that causes delays. Whether or not you've been given a diagnosis for your child's delays, you are probably wondering if there is anything that you can do to help him improve his motor skills. If your child is referred to physical therapy or receives the service, you probably would like to know all about the exercises the therapist does, and why he or she does them. You want to better understand why the physical therapist gives you certain recommendations. What is the purpose of the exercises you are told to do with your child? How will they help him?

This book tries to address these questions. It:

- Focuses on gross motor skills and on how to teach them to your child with the guidance of your physical therapist;
- Explains the intent of common home instructions your therapist may give you;
- Gives you illustrated, easy-to-follow exercise instructions to use with the guidance of your therapist;

- Provides theoretical background information that will increase your knowledge and confidence as you care for your child or talk to various professionals you encounter;
- Deepens your understanding of your own and your physical therapist's contribution to your child's progress.

This book is for parents of children with developmental delay, cerebral palsy, and similar movement disorders who are referred for physical therapy. It explains how your child may learn basic motor skills such as sitting, crawling, standing, and walking with your help and that of the physical therapist. By working together and consistently training missing skills or crucial components of these skills, you and the therapist can help your child reach his fullest potential.

Many illustrated, easy home exercises are presented. Your child's physical or occupational therapist may select the ones best for your child and show you how to use them. Practice these exercises first with the therapist's help and follow any specific instructions the therapist provides. Afterwards, use the exercise routinely, observe the small changes toward progress that may occur, and share them with your therapist. As your child learns a new skill, together you and the therapist will plan how to integrate it into your child's daily life. Implementing this plan will be mostly your job. Examples on how to do this are provided.

Teachers and teaching assistants of children with cerebral palsy and similar movement disorders may find this book equally helpful. Just as parents do, they want to understand their students' physical challenges and help them to achieve their fullest potentials. With creativity and the help of the school physical therapist, they may find ways to adopt some of the home instructions for classroom use. As the children grow and spend more time at school, they will benefit from the integration of their motor skills into their classroom activities.

The book explains terms and concepts that parents or non-medical professionals may encounter. Presented in context, theoretical knowledge educates you about the intent or effect of an exercise. It provides background information and confirms practical advice that will be helpful. For instance, clearly understanding why a muscle needs to be stretched each day or why weight bearing on arms is important makes certain exercises meaningful. Following them may then become more satisfying and motivating.

Treatment narratives explain why some tasks can be so difficult and show how a child may master them. These stories highlight common problems and are meant to deepen the reader's understanding of them. Parents need to be aware that these are mere examples. The problems, as well as the presented solutions, may or may not be applicable to their child.

It is not possible to give specific advice for an individual child in a book. Only the therapist who works with your child and knows his strength and weaknesses—his unique set of problems and his abilities that may help him to overcome them—is in the position to set goals, recommend specific exercises or activities, and give specific instructions.

The information given here is applicable to all children with cerebral palsy and similar movement disorders. They all need help learning basic motor skills. Understanding these skills and how you can help your child acquire them is the emphasis of this text.

Teaching a new motor skill to a child with cerebral palsy or a serious developmental delay is a slow and tedious process. More than thirty years of experience working with children with cerebral palsy has taught me that success depends on the close cooperation and shared expectations of the parent and the therapist. As the story of Nina in the chapter *Head-up* shows, misunderstandings between parent and therapist are not helpful. Working together is the key to success. It assures that your child and his progress remains the focus of the treatment.

It is not easy to raise a child with cerebral palsy and it is not easy to grow up with a disability. It is my wish to help with both.

1
Developmental Delay and Cerebral Palsy

During the first year of life, some babies show a delay in motor development. Later than other children they hold up their head, play with their hands, roll over, sit up, stand, or walk. Premature babies are more likely than other babies to show such a delay. Usually infants with a motor delay are referred to physical therapy. The physical therapists then work with the children and give their parents home instructions. The activities and exercises the therapists and the parents do help the children to learn the missing age-appropriate motor skills. Most infants respond very well to this special help and show good progress with their development.

Some children continue to show very slow progress in spite of the help they receive. They will probably be labeled, at least initially, as having a developmental delay. Developmental delay is a descriptive term. It means that a child's development is slower than that of most children. It does not tell why the child is developing slowly or in what area of development he is delayed. If the children also start to show delays in other areas such as self-feeding, speech, or general responsiveness, they may be called globally delayed. Global delay is also a descriptive term, which does not tell why a child shows this delay in several areas of development.

As children with more serious gross motor delay undergo more testing, they are likely to be specifically diagnosed. Cerebral palsy is one possible diagnosis. There are other diagnoses, which also may be the cause for the delay. Chromosomal abnormalities such as Down syndrome or Prader Willi syndrome, brain malformations such as hydrocephalus or microcephalus, or conditions such as myelination disorders and seizure disorders like infantile spasms are other causes for gross motor delay.

Cerebral Palsy

Cerebral palsy is a disorder of movement and posture. It is caused by a brain injury that occurred before birth, during birth, or during the first few years after birth. The injury hinders the brain's ability to control the muscles of the body properly. The brain tells our muscles how to move and controls the tension of the muscles. Without the proper messages coming from the brain, infants with cerebral palsy have difficulty learning basic motor skills such as crawling, sitting up, or walking.

Since cerebral palsy hinders a child's development and usually causes problems that persist into adulthood, it is classified as a developmental disability. Even though the brain injury that causes cerebral palsy is present at birth, it is often difficult for doctors to recognize it. For this reason, there may be a delay in diagnosis.

How much a child's development is affected by cerebral palsy depends on the extent and location of the brain injury. Different parts of the brain influence our movements in different ways. The damage to the brain may affect some muscles more than others.

Cerebral palsy may be classified either based on the muscles that are most affected or based on the location of the brain injury and the resulting movement problem (Geralis, 1998).

TYPES OF CEREBRAL PALSY

Classifications Based on Muscles Affected

Quadriplegia. This type of cerebral palsy affects the muscles in the child's whole body. The muscles of the trunk, arms, and legs do not work properly. Even the muscles of the face may be affected. This may cause feeding and speech problems in addition to gross and fine motor difficulties. Children with severe quadriplegia have difficulties with most activities of daily living.

Diplegia. Diplegia means that the legs are mainly affected. Often parents do not suspect a problem until their baby is 7 to 9 months old and fails to sit. Typically, children with diplegia gain the coordination and balance required for independent sitting more slowly and not as well as other infants. Standing and walking are affected most. Due to spastic (tight) leg muscles, children with diplegia tend to stand on their toes, turn their legs in, and push their knees together. Depending on the severity of the cerebral palsy, some children with diplegia will be able to walk short distances with a walker, while others may progress to walking independently indoors and then outdoors.

Hemiplegia. In hemiplegia, one side of the body is affected by cerebral palsy. The arm is usually more affected than the leg. Frequently children with hemiplegia are able to compensate for the one-sided disability with their unaffected arm and leg. They may learn most skills almost as quickly as children without cerebral palsy until it is time to walk. Weakness, poor coordination, and spasticity of the affected leg may delay independent walking by a year or more. Depending on the severity of their hemiplegia, the children may have little or limited use of their affected hand.

Classification Based on Location of Brain Injury

Pyramidal (Spastic) Cerebral Palsy. This is the most common type of cerebral palsy. About 80 percent of children with cerebral palsy have spasticity. This means that they have muscles that are tight and limit movements. These children also have involuntary movements caused by abnormal reflexes. See the next chapter for more information on abnormal reflexes.

Extrapyramidal Cerebral Palsy. About 10 percent of children with cerebral palsy have this type of cerebral palsy. They have abnormally low muscle tone, which means that their muscles are weak, and they have difficulty controlling their muscles. These children have involuntary movements, which may include:

- *Athetosis*—the movements are slow and writhing,
- *Ataxia*—the movements are unsteady, shaky, and lack coordination,
- *Dystonia*—the movements are slow, rhythmic, and twisting, or
- *Chorea*—the movements are abrupt, quick, and jerky.

Abnormal movements are discussed in more detail in the next chapter.

Mixed-Type Cerebral Palsy. About 10 percent of children with cerebral palsy have both spastic muscles and the involuntary movements characteristic of extrapyramidal cerebral palsy.

OTHER PROBLEMS RELATED TO CEREBRAL PALSY

The brain injury of the child with cerebral palsy may also affect other areas of the brain. This can cause additional disabilities such as mental retardation, seizure disorder, and vision or hearing loss. Do not assume, however, that your child with cerebral palsy has additional problems. Because a child's movements are different, broadly assuming that other things are wrong does injustice to the child with "only" cerebral palsy.

If your child does turn out to have other disabilities besides cerebral palsy, you will still be able to use the strategies described in this book to help him improve his motor skills. More than likely, however, you will need the assistance of other professionals besides a physical therapist. Depending on his age, your child will qualify for early intervention or special education services that will probably include the services of an infant educator, special education teacher, or other professional who can work with the physical therapist to develop the best methods of teaching your child.

2

Gross Motor Development

Babies are born completely helpless; they have no control over their bodies. Placed on their back, stomach, or side, they will stay there. They have no choice. Even though they do show some organized movement patterns of their head, arms, and legs, these movements are not purposeful and are not controlled voluntarily.

This changes soon after birth as typically developing infants start holding up their head. Thereafter, they reach, kick, roll, crawl, sit, stand, and finally walk. This all happens within approximately one year, which may seem like a long or short period of time, depending on how you look at it. For first-time parents, it may seem endlessly long, and for occasionally visiting grandparents, very short. All these changes that the infant goes through are referred to as gross motor development. Motor means movement. *Gross motor refers to the movements of our big muscles such as the muscles of our shoulders, arms, trunk, hips, or legs.* This is in contrast to fine motor development, which refers to movements of the small muscles of the hand, and oral motor development, which refers to movements of the muscles of the face.

The Sequence of Gross Motor Development

How does gross motor development unfold? As a general guideline *infants acquire motor control "cranial to caudal," meaning from top (the head) to bottom (the hips and legs).* First, children control the muscles of the head, then the shoulders and arms, next the trunk, and last the hips and legs. They develop head to toe. This is good to remember when you observe your child's motor development. It is the same for all developing children, including children with developmental delays or cerebral palsy.

One could compare the first year of motor development to a symphony played by a large orchestra. The music starts softly. Only a few instruments introduce the theme. Soon more instruments join in and the sound becomes full. The music swells and ebbs as different sections of the orchestra show their skills. There are times when all instruments play and it may sound like a big, confusing competition. Yet, at the grand finale they all join together with masterful harmony.

The symphony of an infant's motor development starts with her head. You smile at your baby and show her a pretty rattle. As you move it, she follows it with her eyes and head. Muscles of the neck purposefully turn her head.

A few weeks later you repeat this game. Now you notice that she is also waving her arms. As she excitedly flails them about, she may bat the toy. A week or two later, she may successfully reach for the toy. Clearly, the shoulder and arm muscles are chiming in and trying to work in concert with the muscles of the neck.

Next, as the trunk muscles become active, you will see the first controlled body movement. From side-lying, a typically developing infant rolls to her back or her stomach. When held, she not only holds up her head but also her trunk.

How are her legs and feet doing? Yes, the infant is busily kicking her legs. Purposeful leg movements are seen when she lifts her legs off the floor to touch them or to roll over.

By six months, halfway through the first year of life, a typical baby is using all the big muscles of her body, but has little to show for her efforts. She works hard to sit up, yet topples over quickly. Struggling to move, she manages to circle around on her tummy. Her muscles are not yet well organized. Only her neck muscles have gained good control. She is now holding her head nicely in all positions.

During the following months, the baby masters more important skills. She crawls, pushes into sitting, and sits upright with balance. She happily moves about, plays while sitting, and busily does so all day long. With all of this practice, the muscles of the shoulder and trunk become stronger and more coordinated over time.

Finally, the legs, too, become skilled and strong. The baby practices standing up, coming down, and stepping while holding onto furniture. Then, in a grand finale, all big muscles work together in harmony. The baby takes off and walks.

From now on, mainly the component that had the late start—the hip and leg muscles—and all balance skills will continue to improve for years to come. There is so much more to learn: running, jumping, hopping, skipping, stomping, galloping, standing on one foot, bicycling, and maybe skating or skiing. Balance continues to improve until children are twelve to fifteen years of age (Taguchi and Tada, 1988).

In summary, typically developing children experience a period of fast gross motor development from birth until roughly one year of age followed by a decade of slow further improvement and refinement.

Before addressing how children with cerebral palsy in particular develop, let us pay attention to some lesser known aspects of motor development during the first months of life. It has implications for all children.

The Baby's Position Influences Motor Development

Early motor development occurs in clusters depending on the position the infant is placed in. Infants develop one set of skills in back-lying, another in stomach-lying, and a third when being held in sitting, standing, or being carried. ***How the infant is placed to rest or to play makes a difference.*** When you place your baby on her back, her side, or her stomach, you determine which muscles she will be using. This is just as true for babies with movement disorders such as cerebral palsy as it is for typically developing babies.

Children with cerebral palsy are especially affected by the position they are placed in. They learn to roll over on their own later than other children, and some may never master it. Consequently, the parent or caretaker determines their position.

Knowing how your child's position influences her gross motor development will help you better understand the physical therapist's recommendations. You will know better what to expect when carrying out a home program. It may help you "sneak" little work sessions into your child's daily routine.

BACK-LYING

In back-lying, infants start to use the muscles in front of their body called the flexor muscles. These are the muscles that bend (flex) our joints. When infants hold or move the head in back-lying, the muscles in front of the neck (the neck flexors) are working. They hold their head in the middle or turn it. As a baby gets stronger and more coordinated, she learns to tuck her chin, nod her head, or lift her head off the surface. You may notice your baby craning her head forward in the infant or car seat. She wants to see everything and is using her neck flexors to do so.

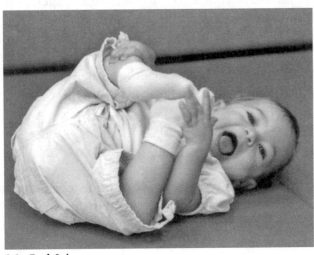

2.1—*Back-Lying.*

Which shoulder muscles are working in back-lying? Again the muscles in front of the shoulder—the shoulder flexors—will bring the arms forward. Bending both shoulder and elbow, the baby brings her hands to her mouth and brings them together over her chest. As these muscles get stronger, she will be able to bring her arms up with elbows straight so that she can reach and play in back-lying.

What else can babies do in back-lying? They kick their legs, they bring their legs up, they touch their knees, and finally they bring their legs up so high and for so long that they can do their favorite thing—play with their feet. Again, the muscles that make this happen are in front of the body. The hip flexors bend the hip and lift the legs up. The tummy muscles (the trunk flexors) help by curling the trunk a little.

Whenever you put your baby on her back, the muscles she uses will be mostly flexor muscles. Therefore, these will become stronger and more coordinated. The same is true when you place your baby in a reclined position, such as in an infant or car seat.

STOMACH-LYING

In stomach-lying, infants start to use the muscles in the back of their body called the extensor muscles. These are the muscles that straighten (extend) the joints.

A newborn baby curls up on her stomach. She looks so uncomfortable with her arms and legs trapped under her body and her head down. The muscles at the back of the neck (the neck extensors) work to lift the head and allow it to turn to the side, so the baby can breathe easier.

The muscles of the back (the shoulder and back extensors) stretch the body and let the arms slide out from under it. The buttock muscles (the hip extensors) stretch out the hip and the baby may lift her legs.

Every time the baby is on her tummy, these muscles are working and getting stronger, yet she accomplishes little. She may lift her head and wave her arms while wiggling her legs, and look like a stranded bird ready for take-off. What a great back strengthening exercise! Try it for yourself. All of her extensor muscles are working.

It takes time for the back muscles to work in coordination with the shoulder and leg muscles. This happens when the baby props herself up on her forearms, or places

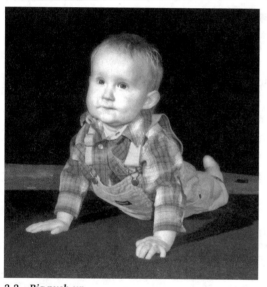

2.2—Big push-up.

her hands on the floor, pushes up, and straightens her elbows (photo 2.2). Now she shifts her weight over one arm as she reaches and plays with the other. While playing on her tummy she learns to move to the side and then also forward. Last she pushes onto hands and knees. From this position she moves into sitting, starts to crawl, and finally pulls to stand.

Whenever you put your baby on her stomach, her neck, shoulder, back, and hip extensor muscles will be working. They will become stronger and more coordinated over time.

The amount of time each day that babies spend on their back, side, or stomach makes a difference. Infants who spend little time on their stomach have less of an opportunity to strengthen their back muscles. Tummy time is especially important for children with cerebral palsy because they usually have weak back muscles. The more chances they have to train these muscles, the better it will be.

OTHER POSITIONS

In side-lying, when held upright, or when moved from one position to another, babies are stimulated to use the flexor and extensor muscles at the same time in sequence or alternately. Whenever you carry your baby, diaper her, change her clothes, or bathe her, you affect her gross motor development. As you roll her from side to side and lift her legs, arms, or head, you trigger muscle responses. Fussing over and playing with your baby is good. It is good for the typically developing child, and it is good for your child with delayed development or cerebral palsy.

Side-lying is a good position for babies to rest or sleep in. When awake, lying on the side makes it easy for infants to bring their hand to their mouth, play with their hands, and look at them. They do not have to lift their arms against gravity as in back-lying. In side-lying, abnormal reflexes and abnormal muscle tone are less likely to interfere with the child's arm movements. For these reasons, your child's physical therapist may recommend side-lying for early arm movements or play activities.

Side-lying is the position infants can move out of easily. An unintentional movement and the pull of gravity will assist them with rolling either onto the stomach or the back. Usually infants first roll out of side-lying incidentally and later discover how to do it purposefully. They learn that bending or straightening the muscles on the side that does not touch the surface will cause the movement out of side-lying. For this reason, babies who are two months or older do not stay in side-lying very long. Within minutes of being placed, they roll out of it.

Positioning in side-lying may be recommended for children with developmental delay or cerebral palsy. Especially for children who are unable to play in back- or stomach-lying, the side position is a good alternative. If your child benefits from being placed in the side position, her therapist will show you ways to prop her up so that she will be able to remain in the position for longer periods of time.

The Motor Development of the Child with Cerebral Palsy

Children with cerebral palsy acquire gross motor skills in the same order as other children. First they hold their head up, then they sit and crawl, and last they walk.

"If this is true," you wonder, "why does my child do everything so differently than other children?" Perhaps you have read about child development in a brochure from the doctor's office or in a book. There were nice pictures showing what babies do at certain ages. Your child does not do these things.

You were told that your child's development would be delayed and that she needs more time than other children to learn basic skills. You are patient and help her along. Your child is growing and learning new things. But, what she does looks different from the pictures in the brochure. What she does may not be shown or mentioned. Therefore, you conclude that your child is not only developing more slowly but also differently from other children.

Your observation is correct. As explained in Chapter 3, differences in your child's muscle tone and in her movement patterns, as well as difficulties controlling her movements, affect her development of motor skills.

Nevertheless, it is also true that children with cerebral palsy usually develop skills in the same sequence as other children. But they acquire skills more slowly and they may learn them in bits and pieces. A skill that babies typically learn within one month may take the child with cerebral palsy two months to learn only partially, and it may take another eight months until she fully masters it. *The initial incomplete skill learning and the following enormous time lag until full mastery of the skill are reasons why the motor development of children with cerebral palsy appears so different.*

Let's use the development of play and reaching in back-lying as an example. The baby in the brochure masters the skill at four months. The child with cerebral palsy may start to play in back-lying around the same time. She may hold a rattle in her hand and purposefully shake it. She may reach, but will not do so in all directions and may not stretch out both arms like the baby in the brochure.

With time and much practice, the child with cerebral palsy may further improve her reaching skill. Finally, she may master it. She stretches both arms forward. But, by then she is no longer a baby who likes to play in back-lying. Instead she sits on her Dad's lap and stretches both arms out, catching the ball Mom rolls to her.

So even though the typically developing baby and the little girl with cerebral palsy do very different activities—one plays with toys dangling from the baby gym while lying on her back and the other plays ball while sitting—both are able to straighten their arms forward. After they have accomplished this skill, they are both ready to put weight on their arms. They are ready to push onto "big arms" with straight elbows, come to hands and knees, and learn to crawl.

ASSESSING DEVELOPMENTAL PROGRESS

With your child developing so differently, what can you expect her to do and when can you expect her to achieve a certain skill? This used to be difficult to answer, because each child with cerebral palsy develops uniquely at her own pace and in her own way. Fortunately, some general guidelines have been developed recently:

- A test to measure the gross motor skills of the children with cerebral palsy has been developed. It is called the *Gross Motor Function Measure* (Russel, 1990). The test tells you what your child can do at the time of testing. Retesting at regular intervals will show your child's progress. The newest version of the test gives you valuable additional information (Russel, 2002). After testing, the physical therapist can show you the items your child passed and other test items in order of difficulty for children with cerebral palsy. The next skills your child may master will most likely be test items of similar difficulty your child has not yet passed. The printout you receive lists the items by title. For a clear understanding of them, ask your physical therapist for an explanation.
- A *Gross Motor Function Classification System for Cerebral Palsy* has been developed. It divides children with cerebral palsy into five different levels, according to their ability, and describes in general terms the gross motor progress of each level between birth and twelve years of age.

Table 2.1 is a reprint of the *Gross Motor Function Classification System* as published by Robert Palisano and colleagues in 1997.

The Gross Motor Function Classification System (GMFCS) and the *Gross Motor Function Measure (GMFM)* have been used by one research team to study the gross motor development of 585 children with cerebral palsy (Palisano, 2000) and by another team to study 657 children with cerebral palsy (Rosenbaum, 2002). The researchers found that the children at all levels made the most progress in motor function between birth and 3 to 4 years of age. By 7 years of age, most of the children had reached their potential. The children at levels IV and V tended to reach their potential earlier than children at levels I, II, or III. The children at level II continued to improve at a slow rate for a longer time than the children at other levels. The first study (Palisano) reports that these children progressed until they were almost 10 years old.

TABLE 2.1	GROSS MOTOR FUNCTION CLASSIFICATION SYSTEM FOR CEREBRAL PALSY

Robert Palisano, Peter Rosenbaum, Stephen Walter, Dianne Russell, Ellen Wood, Barbara Galuppi

INTRODUCTION & USER INSTRUCTIONS

The Gross Motor Function Classification System for cerebral palsy is based on self-initiated movement with particular emphasis on sitting (truncal control) and walking. When defining a 5 level Classification System, our primary criterion was that the distinctions in motor function between levels must be clinically meaningful. Distinctions between levels of motor function are based on functional limitations, the need for assistive technology, including mobility devices (such as walkers, crutches, and canes) and wheeled mobility, and to a much lesser extent quality of movement. Level I includes children with neuromotor impairments whose functional limitations are less than what is typically associated with cerebral palsy, and children who have traditionally been diagnosed as having "minimal brain dysfunction" or "cerebral palsy of minimal severity." The distinctions between Levels I and II therefore are not as pronounced as the distinctions between the other Levels, particularly for infants less than 2 years of age.

The focus is on determining which level best represents the child's present abilities and limitations in motor function. Emphasis is on the child's usual performance in home, school, and community settings. It is therefore important to classify on ordinary performance (not best capacity), and not to include judgments about prognosis. Remember the purpose is to classify a child's present gross motor function, not to judge quality of movement or potential for improvement. The descriptions of the 5 levels are broad and are not intended to describe all aspects of the function of individual children. For example, an infant with hemiplegia who is unable to crawl on hands and knees, but otherwise fits the description of Level I, would be classified in Level I. The scale is ordinal, with no intent that the distances between levels be considered equal or that children with cerebral palsy are equally distributed among the 5 levels. A summary of the distinctions between each pair of levels is provided to assist in determining the level that most closely resembles a child's current gross motor function.

The title for each level represents the highest level of mobility that a child is expected to achieve between 6-12 years of age. We recognize that classification of motor function is dependent on age, especially during infancy and early childhood. For each level, therefore, separate descriptions are provided for children in several age bands. The functional abilities and limitations for each age interval are intended to serve as guidelines, are not comprehensive, and are not norms. Children below age 2 should be considered at their corrected age if they were premature.

An effort has been made to emphasize children's function rather than their limitations. Thus as a general principle, the gross motor function of children who are able to perform the functions described in any particular level will probably be classified at or above that level; in contrast the gross motor functions of children who cannot perform the functions of a particular level will likely be classified below that level.

(Continued on next page.)

(Continued from previous page.)

GROSS MOTOR FUNCTION CLASSIFICATION SYSTEM FOR CEREBRAL PALSY (GMFCS)

Before 2nd Birthday

Level I: Infants move in and out of sitting and floor sit with both hands free to manipulate objects. Infants crawl on hands and knees, pull to stand and take steps holding on to furniture. Infants walk between 18 months and 2 years of age without the need for any assistive mobility device.

Level II: Infants maintain floor sitting but may need to use their hands for support to maintain balance. Infants creep on their stomach or crawl on hands and knees. Infants may pull to stand and take steps holding on to furniture.

Level III: Infants maintain floor sitting when the low back is supported. Infants roll and creep forward on their stomachs.

Level IV: Infants have head control but trunk support is required for floor sitting. Infants can roll to supine and may roll to prone.

Level V: Physical impairments limit voluntary control of movement. Infants are unable to maintain antigravity head and trunk postures in prone and sitting. Infants require adult assistance to roll.

Between 2nd and 4th Birthday

Level I: Children floor sit with both hands free to manipulate objects. Movements in and out of floor sitting and standing are performed without adult assistance. Children walk as the preferred method of mobility without the need for any assistive mobility device.

Level II: Children floor sit but may have difficulty with balance when both hands are free to manipulate objects. Movements in and out of sitting are performed without adult assistance. Children pull to stand on a stable surface. Children crawl on hands and knees with a reciprocal pattern, cruise holding onto furniture and walk using an assistive mobility device as preferred methods of mobility.

Level III: Children maintain floor sitting often by "W-sitting" (sitting between flexed and internally rotated hips and knees) and may require adult assistance to assume sitting. Children creep on their stomach or crawl on hands and knees (often without reciprocal leg movements) as their primary methods of self-mobility. Children may pull to stand on a stable surface and cruise short distances. Children may walk short distances indoors using an assistive mobility device and adult assistance for steering and turning.

Level IV: Children floor sit when placed, but are unable to maintain alignment and balance without use of their hands for support. Children frequently require adaptive equipment for sitting and standing. Self-mobility for short distances (within a room) is achieved through rolling, creeping on stomach, or crawling on hands and knees without reciprocal leg movement.

Level V: Physical impairments restrict voluntary control of movement and the ability to maintain antigravity head and trunk postures. All areas of motor function are limited. Functional limitations in sitting and standing are not fully compensated for through the use of adaptive equipment and assistive technology. At Level V, children have no means of independent mobility and are transported. Some children achieve self-mobility using a power wheelchair with extensive adaptations.

Between 4th and 6th Birthday

Level I: Children get into and out of, and sit in, a chair without the need for hand support. Children move from the floor and from chair sitting to standing without the need for objects for support. Children walk indoors and outdoors, and climb stairs. Emerging ability to run and jump.

Level II: Children sit in a chair with both hands free to manipulate objects. Children move from the floor to standing and from chair sitting to standing but often require a stable surface to push or pull up on with their arms. Children walk without the need for any assistive mobility device indoors and for short distances on level surfaces outdoors. Children climb stairs holding onto a railing but are unable to run or jump.

Level III: Children sit on a regular chair but may require pelvic or trunk support to maximize hand function. Children move in and out of chair sitting using a stable surface to push on or pull up with their arms. Children walk with an assistive mobility device on level surfaces and climb stairs with assistance from an adult. Children frequently are transported when travelling for long distances or outdoors on uneven terrain.

Level IV: Children sit on a chair but need adaptive seating for trunk control and to maximize hand function. Children move in and out of chair sitting with assistance from an adult or a stable surface to push or pull up on with their arms. Children may at best walk short distances with a walker and adult supervision but have difficulty turning and maintaining balance on uneven surfaces. Children are transported in the community. Children may achieve self-mobility using a power wheelchair.

Level V: Physical impairments restrict voluntary control of movement and the ability to maintain antigravity head and trunk postures. All areas of motor function are limited. Functional limitations in sitting and standing are not fully compensated for through the use of adaptive equipment and assistive technology. At Level V, children have no means of independent mobility and are transported. Some children achieve self-mobility using a power wheelchair with extensive adaptations.

Between 6th and 12th Birthday

Level I: Children walk indoors and outdoors, and climb stairs without limitations. Children perform gross motor skills including running and jumping but speed, balance, and coordination are reduced.

Level II: Children walk indoors and outdoors, and climb stairs holding onto a railing but experience limitations walking on uneven surfaces and inclines, and walking in crowds or confined spaces. Children have at best only minimal ability to perform gross motor skills such as running and jumping.

Level III: Children walk indoors or outdoors on a level surface with an assistive mobility device. Children may climb stairs holding onto a railing. Depending on upper limb function, children propel a wheelchair manually or are transported when traveling for long distances or outdoors on uneven terrain.

Level IV: Children may maintain levels of function achieved before age 6 or rely more on wheeled mobility at home, school, and in the community. Children may achieve self-mobility using a power wheelchair.

(Continued on next page.)

(Continued from previous page.)

Level V: Physical impairments restrict voluntary control of movement and the ability to maintain antigravity head and trunk postures. All areas of motor function are limited. Functional limitations in sitting and standing are not fully compensated for through the use of adaptive equipment and assistive technology. At level V, children have no means of independent mobility and are transported. Some children achieve self-mobility using a power wheelchair with extensive adaptations.

DISTINCTIONS BETWEEN LEVELS I AND II

Compared with children in Level I, children in Level II have limitations in the ease of performing movement transitions; walking outdoors and in the community; the need for assistive mobility devices when beginning to walk; quality of movement; and the ability to perform gross motor skills such as running and jumping.

DISTINCTIONS BETWEEN LEVELS II AND III

Differences are seen in the degree of achievement of functional mobility. Children in Level III need assistive mobility devices and frequently orthoses to walk, while children in Level II do not require assistive mobility devices after age 4.

DISTINCTIONS BETWEEN LEVEL III AND IV

Differences in sitting ability and mobility exist, even allowing for extensive use of assistive technology. Children in Level III sit independently, have independent floor mobility, and walk with assistive mobility devices. Children in Level IV function in sitting (usually supported) but independent mobility is very limited. Children in Level IV are more likely to be transported or use power mobility.

DISTINCTIONS BETWEEN LEVELS IV AND V

Children in Level V lack independence even in basic antigravity postural control. Self-mobility is achieved only if the child can learn how to operate an electrically powered wheelchair.

Reference: *Developmental Medicine & Child Neurology 1997; 39*:214-223.

© 1997 CanChild Centre for Childhood Disability Research (formerly NCRU), McMaster University, Hamilton, ON, Canada L8S 1C7; www.fhs.mcmaster.ca/canchild

The authors of the studies believe that the GMFCS and GMFM provide valuable information to parents of children with cerebral palsy and to professionals working with the children. They give general guidelines concerning the gross motor progress and potential of the children. However, the authors state: "This information may be useful in anticipating change over time *but should not be used to predict the future gross motor function for an individual child.*" They recommend that the information be used in conjunction with other relevant information when making decisions concerning a specific child.

Frequently Asked Questions

Q. *"You talked about how different positions affect babies. Is the same true for older children?"*

A. Yes, for example, a child who mostly sits in a reclined position or lies on her back will not exercise her back muscles.

Q. *"I want Megan to sit by herself. How does the Gross Motor Function Measure tell me when she will do this?"*

A. The Gross Motor Function Measure does not tell you when Megan may sit. The chart that accompanies the test gives general guidelines. For instance, it tells you which test items most children master before they sit on their own on a bench for 10 seconds.

Q. *"Dustin is five years old. His physical therapist told us that Dustin is at level III of the Gross Motor Function Classification System. Does that mean that he will not walk? We are very upset about this."*

A. I understand your feelings. Who wouldn't be if told that their child may need a walker or crutches for walking? Your reaction shows how much you love Dustin.

Remember that the Gross Motor Function Classification System gives only general guidelines. Do not give up hope too early. You have nothing to lose when working with him toward independent standing and walking. The training will be valuable even if Dustin ultimately does not succeed in walking without some support. The balance and coordination he gains will make walking with support easier and more efficient. This means that his endurance will improve. Also, when Dustin becomes really comfortable with his walker or crutches they may bother him less than you may think. I have seen quite a few happy smiles on the faces of children who walked with assistive devices.

Q. *"Wouldn't it be better not to know my child's level and all the information about it?"*

A. I don't have a good answer to this. This is new information and time will tell how helpful it is. I believe, however, that the information is very valuable for parents of older children with cerebral palsy. It confirms when their child has reached her fullest potential.

3

Obstacles to Motor Development

The previous chapter touched on two of the effects that cerebral palsy has on a child's muscles. It causes problems with muscle tone and also with involuntary or abnormal movements. This chapter focuses in more detail on how differences in muscle tone, as well as abnormal movement patterns or reflexes can complicate the acquisition of motor skills.

Muscle Tone

What is muscle tone? Muscle tone refers to the amount of tension or resistance to movement within a muscle. Muscles have elastic properties, similar to a rubber band. Rubber bands are soft or hard, depending on how easily they are stretched. Muscles have low or high tone, which makes them easy or less easy to stretch.

Muscle tone varies from person to person. Some people have low muscle tone. Their muscles are soft, have little tension, and are easily stretched. Other people have higher muscle tone. More resistance is felt when their muscles are stretched. Even when resting, their muscles are somewhat taut and have more tension.

Children with cerebral palsy have muscle tone that is outside the normal variation. If the tone is very low it is called hypotonic or flaccid. *A hypotonic or flaccid muscle is soft and very stretchable.* There is hardly any resistance felt when an arm or leg is moved.

If the tone is very high it is called hypertonic or spastic. *A hypertonic or spastic muscle feels hard and resists being stretched.* If the spastic muscle is stretched slowly, the same amount of resistance is felt until the muscle is stretched to its full length. But if you stretch the same muscle quickly, the resistance increases and stops the movement before the muscle reaches its full length.

Children with cerebral palsy may have hypertonic muscles or hypotonic muscles, or a combination of both types of muscle tone. Children with milder forms of cerebral palsy may have a combination of muscles with normal and abnormal tone. Some children have fluctuating muscle tone. This means that the tone of a muscle swings from being very low at rest to very high when the muscle works. At birth, however, most children with cerebral palsy have low muscle tone. Often, it is not until many months later that the first signs of abnormal high muscle tone are seen, and additional months pass before a diagnosis of cerebral palsy is confirmed.

Muscle tone is regulated by nerve cells in our brain. Children with cerebral palsy have damage to those nerve tissues. Which parts of their bodies are affected and how much they are affected by abnormal muscle tone depends upon where and how much damage has occurred in the brain.

Your child's muscle tone affects his movements and motor development. Hypotonia—very low muscle tone—makes it harder for children to move against gravity, resistance and to move forcefully. In stomach-lying, for instance, it is difficult for them to push off, straighten the elbow, and raise their chest off the floor. After much practice, as the children get stronger and more coordinated, the effect of the low muscle tone will become less noticeable.

Hypertonicity—very high muscle tone—means that children have to work very hard to overcome the resistance of spastic and tense muscles. For instance, if the inner thigh muscles are spastic, they will pull the leg inward. When the child wants to move his legs outward, he must overcome the tension of these spastic muscles. Depending on the child's position and the task at hand, this may be easier in some situations than in others. The exercises and activities your therapist recommends and the ones given in this book try to minimize the influence of the spastic muscles.

The abnormal muscle tone caused by cerebral palsy is not progressive. In other words, it will not get worse over the course of your child's life. It also will not get better. Your child will not "grow out" of his muscle tone problems, nor will exercises help normalize his tone. ***However, therapeutic exercises and activities will help him master motor skills in spite of his abnormal muscle tone.*** And, as discussed later in the book, exercises and stretching are very important in preventing complications such as joint contractions that can make movement more difficult.

Muscle tone is affected by emotions. You may already know this from experience. You quiver with joy or are frozen by fear so that you stiffen your neck and back. The same happens to children with cerebral palsy, only much more so. They literally may fall down laughing or go to pieces crying.

Strong emotions bring about an abnormal increase of muscle tone in children with cerebral palsy. They may lose control of their muscles, and abnormal movement patterns are more likely to occur. For this reason it is best to keep excitement—good or bad—to a minimum when you work with your child on motor skills.

Yes, you want to motivate your child to roll over onto his tummy. Encourage him, but don't cheer him on as he goes about it. Excitement increases his muscle tone and may cause him to tumble onto his back again.

Loud sounds and bright lights may also affect muscle tone. If this is so for your child, avoid both when you work with him.

Abnormal Movement Patterns

Children with cerebral palsy may exhibit not only abnormal muscle tone but also abnormal movement patterns. A movement pattern is a sequence of movements. When we use our muscles, we usually do not make one single movement but a sequence of movements. For instance, when we take a step, turn around, or shake hands, we use a movement pattern to do these things.

When a child with spastic quadriplegic cerebral palsy wants to reach and grasp something, the following may happen: the arm comes up, but instead of straightening, the elbow bends; instead of turning out, the arm turns in; instead of straightening, the wrist twists; and instead of opening, the hand fists or curls.

It is not that the child wants to make this abnormal movement. If you tell him to try harder and do a better job, most likely the outcome will even be worse. The extra effort will increase the tension of the child's hypertonic muscles. This in turn can make the resulting movement even more abnormal.

Children with athetoid cerebral palsy show involuntary arm and leg movements even when they want to stand still. Reaching for an object, their hands may move beyond the target. When they walk, their body and arms may move so much that they have difficulty keeping their balance.

The abnormal extension pattern of the legs is one of the most frequently occurring atypical movement patterns in children with cerebral palsy. It is called scissoring. Even children with mild cerebral palsy may show this pattern when they are first standing. They stand on their toes with stiff legs, which are turned inward and pushed together. If children walk this way, their legs cross over with each step (hence the name scissoring). Many children with cerebral palsy show only some features of the pattern. Children may soon learn to keep their legs apart, even though they may still stand on their toes.

COMBINED NORMAL AND ABNORMAL MOVEMENT PATTERNS

Children with moderate or mild cerebral palsy most likely will not show full abnormal movement patterns. Instead they may use a variation of normal movements combined with some abnormal features. For example, a child may only partially stretch his elbow and partially open his hand during reaching. Why this is so is not fully understood. Fortunately, we know from experience that the motor pattern, in this case reaching, does improve with therapy and training.

Reflexes

Abnormal reflexes may cause some of the abnormal movements we see in children with cerebral palsy. Reflexes are involuntary movements that occur in response to a stimulus such as touch, pressure, or joint movement. Most reflexes are helpful. For example, when something is stuck in your throat, the coughing or gag reflex helps you to remove it quickly.

There are some reflexes that only occur in infants during the first months of life and then they fade away. They are called primitive reflexes and are normal. In children with cerebral palsy, these reflexes may persist and may be more pronounced. They are then called atypical or abnormal.

ABNORMAL REFLEXES COMMON IN CEREBRAL PALSY

Depending on the severity and type of cerebral palsy, there may be several types of abnormal reflex patterns, including:

1. the tonic labyrinthine reflex,
2. asymmetrical tonic neck reflex,
3. symmetrical tonic neck reflex,
4. startle reflex.

The first two are more likely to occur in children with more severe cerebral palsy, and can cause major problems. (Bobath, 1980). These reflexes are most likely to occur when the children lie on their backs.

Tonic Labyrinthine Reflex. When lying on the back, the tonic labyrinthine reflex causes the muscle tone of back muscles to increase. The child's back straightens or even curves backwards. The legs are straight, stiff, pushed together or crossed, and the feet are pointed. The arms are bent at the elbows. The wrists are bent and the hand is fisted or the fingers are curled. This reflex is also referred to as abnormal extension pattern or extensor tone.

Asymmetrical Tonic Neck Reflex (ATNR). When children with severe cerebral palsy push their head back and turn it sharply to one side, this will trigger another abnormal pattern. The arm on the face side stretches out, the other arm bends at the elbow, and the legs show a corresponding pattern of one leg straight and the other bent.

The tonic labyrinthine and the asymmetrical tonic neck reflex patterns are totally useless. They hinder functional activities such as rolling, bringing the hands together, or even bringing the hands to the mouth. Over time, the reflex patterns can cause serious damage to the growing child's joints and bones. The ATNR may twist the spine into a curvature (scoliosis). Both the tonic labyrinthine reflex and the ATNR may cause the head of the thighbone to slip partially out of the hip socket (hip subluxation). Or the head of the thighbone may move completely out of the socket (hip dislocation).

For these reasons, a back-lying position may need to be avoided for a child who has these persistent reflexes. Fortunately, it is less likely that the abnormal reflexes will occur and affect the child's muscle tone in other positions such as side-lying, reclined sitting, or straight sitting. If they do, they are not as strong, and are less likely to affect the whole body. Even for young children with milder forms of cerebral palsy, who show little progress with "happy baby" activities (See Chapter 7), it is best not to have them lie on their backs for long periods of time when they are awake.

In addition, parents of children with cerebral palsy are told not to carry their child with the trunk and legs all straight, because a backwards movement of the child's head may trigger the extension reflex pattern. Instead, parents are advised to snuggle the child close to their body with both or one leg bent.

As another preventive measure, all small children at risk of, or diagnosed with, cerebral palsy should be discouraged from pushing their head back and turning it far to one side. Even if the child does not show an ATNR reflex pattern, the position of the head and neck changes the muscle tone in the arms and makes it harder for the child to use them. It is always best if your child's head is in the middle and faces forward. When your child starts to play with his hands and feet in back-lying, this precaution may be disregarded.

Symmetrical Tonic Neck Reflex (STNR). A third abnormal reflex that may be seen in children with cerebral palsy is called the symmetrical tonic neck reflex (STNR). When the head is extended, the STNR causes the arms to straighten and the legs to bend. When the head is bent, the STNR causes the arms to bend and the legs to straighten. The reflex may assist the child to come to a bunny position. Yet, when the child is ready to crawl on hands and knees, the reflex may cause him to "bunny hop" and hinder the development of a reciprocal crawl (in which the left arm and right leg move forward, followed by the right arm and left leg).

Startle Reflex. Some children with cerebral palsy are very easily startled by sudden noises or events. A door opening, a dog barking, someone calling, or the telephone ringing may cause these children to startle. The startle reaction sharply increases the children's muscle tone. Muscle control decreases, and, as a result, the children may momentarily lose their balance and fall.

For some parents, their child's startle reflex is a constant concern. Safety features of adapted chairs or standers address this problem. Your child's physical therapist will assist you in finding the right equipment for your child.

In summary, the degree to which abnormal reflexes hinder a child's development varies greatly. The more persistent and pronounced these abnormal reflexes patterns are, the more they interfere with learning useful movements such as reaching, crawling, or walking, as well as positions such as sitting, kneeling, and standing. Parents of children with cerebral palsy want to avoid triggering abnormal reflexes. They can do this by following the general guidelines mentioned here and the specific advice they are receiving from their child's therapist.

Lack of Motor Control and Coordination

The inability to control the muscles is the most pervasive problem of children with cerebral palsy and similar movement disorders. This lack of control is most obvious if a child has spasticity. In the past, it was believed that hypertonicity *caused* the lack of muscle control. It is true that spasticity interferes with muscle control. Yet, it is not its cause. Muscle control problems are present independent of muscle tone issues. That is why medicine, which reduces high muscle tone, will not automatically improve the child's muscle control. Children with cerebral palsy and similar movement disorders who have hypotonia also have difficulty with muscle control.

What exactly is muscle control? Muscle control allows us to use our muscles and move our body as we want to. It allows us to regulate the force, speed, and timing of our movements. A gymnast who does a graceful forward roll or back flip shows very good muscle control and coordination. No one expects that a small child will do something like this. Yet, even when a baby sits or stands up, he controls the force, speed, and timing of his muscles. A baby may first sit up clumsily. As he does it again and again his movements may become smooth. We may say that he sits up with good coordination. Typically, children develop muscle control and coordination as they grow up.

Children with cerebral palsy have less muscle control. They have difficulty moving strongly or lightly, quickly or slowly, or sequencing and timing their movements. Instead of moving one leg, they may move both legs; instead of lightly taking a plastic cup, they may grab it with too much force and crush it; instead of quickly stretching their arms to catch a ball, they may move too slowly and miss it. The children show improvement of muscle control and coordination with therapy and training, unless they have very significant disabilities.

Muscle Weakness

Children with cerebral palsy and similar movement disorders also lack muscle strength and endurance. If a child has low muscle tone, the lack of strength is very obvious. When lying on his stomach, the child may be too weak to lift his head and push up with his arms. As he improves, he may push up for a short time. He lacks the endurance to push up longer. After more practice, he slowly will get stronger and becomes able to hold up his head and push off with his arms for a longer time.

Muscle weakness is also present in children with high tone. A spastic muscle feels hard and tense. Therefore, you may believe the muscle to be strong. However, the muscle may be weak. The latest research indicates, in fact, that spasticity and strength are not interrelated (Ross and Engsberg, 2002). Frequently the spastic muscle and the muscle opposing it are both weak and need to be strengthened. This can be done. Previously it was believed that strengthening would harm the spastic muscles and that their muscle tone would become even more spastic by strengthening. New research proves otherwise (Fowler, 2001).

How much a lack of muscle strength interferes with a child's motor development varies. Usually, however, slow progress is caused by problems with muscle control and not by weakness.

Abnormal Sensory Awareness

Children with cerebral palsy may have an injury to the part of the brain, which interprets sensory information from the senses of touch, positioning, and movement. As a result, children may be hypo- or hypersensitive. A child with hyposensitivity to touch receives little information when touching something or when being touched. The reduced sense of touch will make it harder for him to use his hands. Imagine that you are wearing gloves as you grasp something or try to tie a knot. The gloves reduce the sensory information you receive and make the job harder. A child with hyposensitivity to touch may be in a similar situation.

Children who receive less information than usual from their feet and their sense of position have trouble feeling where their feet are and how much pressure they exert on the ground. Their situation may be similar to what you experience when you stand in deep water and the information you receive from your feet is rather vague so that standing still is more difficult than on land.

Children with hypersensitivity receive too much information. For this reason, touching something or being touched may be unpleasant and these children may avoid both. A child may receive more information than usual from his sense of position when he puts weight on his feet as he stands or on his hands as he crawls. This hypersensitivity makes it unpleasant and uncomfortable to bear weight, so children try to avoid it.

Chapter 9 describes how abnormal sensory awareness interferes with a child's motor development and shows how he gradually overcomes this obstacle.

4

Helping Your Child Learn Motor Skills

If you have read the preceding chapters, you may be wondering how it is possible for children with cerebral palsy or similar movement disorders to master the gross motor skills they need. If their difficulties with muscle tone, abnormal movement patterns, lack of motor control, muscle weakness, abnormal sensory awareness, and slowed development are due to a brain injury or a developmental defect of the central nervous system, what can help them overcome these problems? There are two answers:

1. The brain can, to a certain extent, recover from, or compensate, for injury, and
2. Parents and therapists can teach children the most effective ways to learn and practice motor skills.

Neural Plasticity

At birth, an infant's brain is not fully developed. During the first and second year of life, the brain is still growing, changing, and forming new connections. Therefore, it is possible that other cells may take over the work of the damaged cells. With stimulation and training, this is more likely to happen. This capacity of the brain to adapt to, and supplement for, a deficit is called neural plasticity.

As brain growth subsides, neural plasticity decreases. New research, however, indicates that some capacity for recovery remains throughout a person's life. Even if an adult suffers an injury to her central nervous system, other nerve cells may take over all or part of the function of the damaged cells. Special training as soon as possible after the injury makes this more likely.

Physical Therapy Treatment and Motor Learning

Another possible way children with cerebral palsy may acquire a basic skill such as crawling or sitting up is by training. How this training is done has evolved over the years. There are several sources of information that guide therapists when they work with children or advise their parents, caretakers, or teachers. One is a rapidly expanding body of knowledge called motor learning. The other sources are concepts and techniques developed by professionals intimately familiar with the characteristics, problems, and potentials of children with cerebral palsy or similar movement disorders.

Motor Learning

Physical education teachers, athletic trainers, and coaches specialize in teaching children and adults a great variety of motor skills we call sports. Children learn to swim, skate, dance, ski, horseback ride, do gymnastics, play tennis, and so on. They are not born with the ability to perform these sports. It is exposure to and training of the skills that lead to their mastery.

How quickly and how well a person learns a new sport depends on many factors. Aptitude, motivation, and opportunities for practice are important. But how well a sport is taught also plays a significant role. Scientists have been investigating how people learn a new motor skill and how to teach them best. As they asked questions, tested, got answers, and arrived at conclusions, they gained new insights and understandings. A whole field of study developed—the science of motor learning.

The knowledge of motor learning pertains to how a healthy person learns a physical skill. Does this knowledge apply to people with a neurological deficit? Does it apply to children with cerebral palsy? Some studies have tried to answer this question (Thorpe & Valvano, 2002). So far, there is no clear answer. Yet, at this time the general consensus is that insights gained in the field of motor learning may also explain how children with cerebral palsy learn basic motor skills (Shumway-Cook & Woollacott, 2001). The following section presents some of the findings.

PRINCIPLES OF MOTOR LEARNING TO KEEP IN MIND

1. Learning a new motor skill is an active process.

It involves finding an efficient, consistent solution to a motor problem. What does this mean? Let's use an example—your child is able to sit but is unable to get down from sitting. The motor problem she has to solve is how to move from sitting to the floor with ease and control. For a small child, the best way to do this is to turn to the side and place both hands on the floor. With her arms in a good position to guide her movements and soften the impact, she may now lower her trunk and slides down on her belly without getting hurt. The therapist will show you how to help your child perform this movement sequence. As you follow the instructions at home, your child will get acquainted with the movement pattern and her arm muscles may get stronger as she bears weight on them. But true skill learning will only happen if your child also participates with problem solving. When your child wants to move (there is a toy on the floor she likes to play with), gets only some help from you, and does as much as possible on her own, then she takes part in the problem solving process and skill learning happens.

2. Motivation is an important part of skill learning.

Therefore, before you practice a skill with your child, look for ways to motivate her. For instance, when your child is happily sitting and playing, it is not a good time to practice moving down to the floor. She will not be motivated to do so. Instead, wait until she is done playing and ready to get to the interesting toy you placed on the floor. Only if she wants to be on the floor will she be motivated to learn and try to perform the movement sequence of lowering herself out of sitting. Learning does not take place without motivation.

3. Active exploration helps skill learning.

The more a child is allowed to actively explore and find solutions to motor problems, the more skills she will learn and the better she will learn them. You may believe that helping your child to move perfectly and smoothly from sitting to the floor will enhance good learning. This is not true. Padding the floor with an extra rug and allowing your child to do as much as possible on her own will further motor learning. Her movements may be choppy, and lack grace and fluency as she struggles on her own. Yet, do not worry; she will be learning. Motor skill learning requires many repetitions before you may expect efficiency and smoothness. You have to remember how often you had to bat a baseball or do a golf stroke before you got good at it.

4. A demonstration may help your child.

A sibling may model for your child how to do a movement such as getting down from sitting or you may show her using a doll. If you do, emphasize the outcome of the movement sequence—in our example, it would be sliding onto the belly and reaching the toy. Researchers found that this is the way children learn best. Also, modeling a new skill smoothly and perfectly is not as helpful to a beginning learner as watching someone struggle to perform the skill.

5. Variability helps skill learning.

Initially, your consistent help will make it easier for your child to perform a new movement sequence. As soon as your child improves, however, vary your approach. Try not to always help her in the very same way. Do not always place the toy she wants to get to in the very same spot. The more variable the practice, the better your child will learn the new skill.

6. Practice a skill until it is well learned.

Just because your child successfully moved from sitting to her tummy once does not mean she has mastered the skill. Encourage her to practice until the skill is well learned. Only after a skill is well learned will your child always be able to do it. If it is not well learned, she may lose it again. When your child moves from sitting to the floor with ease and does so on her own during play, this skill is well learned. It is now part of her skill repertoire.

7. Transfer of learning may occur.

Transfer of learning means that learning one skill may help your child to learn another skill. When and how much transfer of learning occurs is important to know. Researchers found that the better a skill is learned and the more variably it is practiced, the more likely transfer of learning will happen. Also, the more alike two skills are, the more likely it is for transfer of learning to occur. For instance, if a child learns to move from sitting to the floor well, she may learn to push into sitting from being on the floor fairly quickly there-after. Moving into sitting and moving out of sitting are two skills that share movement components. Therefore, mastery of one skill will help a child learn the other.

8. Some skills may have negative transfer effects.

A two-year-old child may teach herself to move from sitting to the floor by slowly rolling backwards. Doing so will not have a positive transfer effect in regard to moving into sitting. That is, it will not help her learn a related skill. If she tries to sit up using the same motor pattern she used rolling down, she will not succeed. It is only between 68 and 72 months of age that a typically developing child is able to sit up this way (Peabody Developmental Motor Scale, 2000). A child with cerebral palsy will not be able to do it any earlier. On the other hand, going down and sitting up by placing both hands forward and sideways is mastered by typically developing children between 7 to 9 months of age. Consequently, children with cerebral palsy are more likely to become successful when they use this same pattern.

9. Similar motor skills may need to be learned separately.

Research indicates that we learn motor skills more specifically than once was assumed. For instance, you may think that sitting on a chair and sitting on the floor are one and the same skill. In both situations the person sits, so it may be assumed that when she learns to sit, she becomes able to sit either on the floor or in a chair. In fact, this may not be true. Sitting on a chair and sitting on a floor may be two separate skills. To master them, both may have to be trained.

Specificity of learning and transfer of learning are interrelated concepts. At this time we do not yet know how they apply to many practical situations. Future research should tell us.

10. Feedback helps skill learning.

Through feedback, the child receives information about how she performed a task. Feedback may come in many forms. When your child moves from sitting on the floor to stomach-lying, she perceives how it feels to turn her body slightly to the side, put weight on her arms, bend her arms, and touch the floor with her belly. She will notice if she is able to reach the toy she wants to play with. She will see her parents' smiling faces and hear their applause as she succeeds. All of this is helpful feedback.

Most parents like to give verbal feedback. They like to encourage and praise their children. Researchers asked the question of how often verbal feedback should be given. They found that steady verbal feedback is not as effective as intermittent feedback. Especially initially, verbal feedback may distract children from the task and may let them pay less attention to the feedback they receive from their senses. So, if you feel the urge to talk to and encourage your child, relax and do it only every once and a while. On the other hand, a loving smile or approving nod should always be helpful.

11. Don't ask your child to show off a new skill too soon.

Researchers investigated the audience effect. They found that well-learned skills become better in front of an audience but a new skill may deteriorate. This explains why your child may not be able to demonstrate her newest trick to her grandparents or the therapist. After more practice, as the new skill becomes firmer, this should change.

12. The more practice, the better.

The more practice you can provide for your child, the more she learns. This makes sense, and motor learning research has confirmed it.

How much should you practice a skill with your child? Should you practice with her moving from sitting to the floor one time, then give her some free time, and later practice again? Or should you practice lots of time in a row with little rest in between? If you practice crawling with your child, should you take care that she practices only a short distance or should you encourage her to continue crawling as far as she possibly can? Researchers have looked into this. They found that it is all right to practice the same task again and again with little rest in between. They call it **massed practice.** Even if a person got tired after many repetitions and did not do the task as well as before, researchers found that learning occurred. In fact, at times massed practice brings better learning than practice distributed over a longer period of time.

After a child has initially been reluctant to practice a new skill, it frequently happens that suddenly she really likes to practice. Whenever this happens, let your child practice as much as she wants to—you know she is learning. If, after many repetitions, she gets tired and does not do as well as before—you know she is still learning. You may have to watch her more closely for safety reasons, however. And don't forget to praise and hug her afterwards. (Not in between, as that would interfere with her learning.)

13. Ask the therapist how often to practice with your child each week.

The optimal amount of time to practice exercises depends on the type of exercise. Stretching exercises have to be done every day. Fortunately, stretching does not take much time. Depending on how many stretches your child needs, a stretching program may be done in less than 5 to 15 minutes. (See Chapter 5 for information on stretching.) Strengthening exercises are effective if done three to four times a week. Skill and balance training does not have to be done on a specific schedule. Yet time on task matters. More practice will bring about more learning. If in doubt about the frequency and length of practice sessions, be sure to ask your child's physical therapist.

Physical Therapy for Children with Cerebral Palsy

Decades ago, before scientists started studying treatment outcomes, therapists learned from their experience—from their successes and failures—how to help children with cerebral palsy and similar movement disorders. Experienced therapists with a keen sense of observation and insight shared their experience and advanced the treatment. One of these therapists was Bertha Bobath. Fifty years ago, while working in a London hospital, Mrs. Bobath noted the difficulties her patients had as she treated them lying on their backs in their beds—as was customary in this hospital at the time. Compassionate, gifted, and energetic, Mrs. Bobath instead placed the children in different positions and supported and assisted them with her large, strong hands. While Mrs. Bobath worked with the children, they were able to hold their head or move their arms in ways they had not been able to before. Delighted, she shared her observations with her husband, Karel, a physician. Together they developed a new way of treating children with cerebral palsy called Neurodevelopmental Treatment (NDT).

The Bobaths devoted the rest of their lives to improving and refining their treatment method and taught it to therapists all over the world. Many therapeutic techniques that therapists use today were first advocated by Bertha Bobath. But some of the NDT principles had to be changed or were replaced as sciences advanced.

It is not the intent of this book to describe the NDT treatment or any other treatment approach. Instead the following tries to summarize treatment components understood as best practice in providing physical therapy treatment of children with cerebral palsy and similar movement disorders.

BEARING WEIGHT WITH GOOD POSTURE

Bearing weight—putting weight on your arms or legs—encourages the muscles to work. When you lean on your arms and the weight of your upper body bears down on them, your arm and shoulder muscles work to hold you up. When you stand and the weight of your body bears down, your leg, hip, and back muscles work to hold you up. Therapists use this response to strengthen the muscles of children with hypotonia. Even if a child is too weak to hold herself up, assisted weight bearing is beneficial for her. Her effort to stand or hold herself up with her arms has a strengthening effect.

In children with hypertonicity, weight bearing may bring about an extremely strong response. The children may stiffly straighten their arms or legs. All their muscles respond instead of just the ones needed to hold themselves up. This type of reaction to weight bearing is not helpful. When the arms are stiffly straightened, the child cannot bend her elbows. Yet, bending the arms is necessary—for instance, when the child sits on the floor, props on her arms, and wants to lower herself onto her tummy. Likewise, when the child stands with stiffly straightened legs, she cannot bend her knees or her ankles. Therefore, she cannot sit down or walk.

Therapists discovered that when children with cerebral palsy weight bear with a good posture, they show a more normal muscle response. When bearing weight on their arms, therapists helped the children to place their open hands down and support their shoulders in a good position so they were not pulled up or back. They placed the hand, elbow, and shoulder joints in alignment. Now the arm muscles response became more normal. With training, the children could learn to bend the elbows with control, shift their weight over one arm, and so on.

When the therapists help the children to stand with feet flat on the floor, toes pointing forward or slightly outward, hips and trunk straight or slightly tilted forward, the children no longer stiffened their legs. Instead of all their muscles responding at once, they began to use mostly the muscles needed to hold themselves up. With consistent training they could now bend their knees a little and straighten them again, shift most of their weight onto one leg, and so on.

Weight bearing with good posture can be done in many different positions—on hands and knees, propped on elbows, and in side leaning, side sitting, squatting, kneeling, half-kneeling, half standing, and more. It is an important tool. It improves strength and coordination. Depending on the position, it also stretches specific muscles. Therapists teach bearing weight with a good posture to parents and professionals working with the children. The illustrated weight bearing activities in this book should make the task easier.

CONTROLLED WEIGHT SHIFT

The ability of shifting weight means that you move your body weight from one part of your body to another. Trying to tap dance is an easy way to experience weight shift. You stand, move your body weight over one foot, and than tap with the other foot. As you take turns tapping with the right and then the left foot, you will notice how you shift your weight before each tap. Watch someone else tap dance and you can easily observe her shift her weight. Frequently you shift your weight without noticing it. You may be surprised to learn that all movements entail some weight shifts. The weight shifts are often very small and subtle. You only shift as much as needed. This way you remain stable and balanced as you move. The more fine-tuned your weight shifts are, the more fluent and coordinated your movements are.

Uncontrolled weight shifts produce jerky movements. A person who cannot control her weight shifts in standing will lose her balance and fall.

Children first learn to shift their weight when lying on the floor. The skill that most obviously involves weight shifts is rolling. Once children are able to roll over on their own they frequently enjoy the activity. They may teach themselves to roll and roll—thereby traveling on the floor wherever they want to go.

When the children sit up they slowly learn to control weight shifts and balance in sitting. In the beginning your child will sit very quietly on the floor. You want to reinforce this. As she quietly plays, she learns to control small weight shifts. Small and slow weight shifts are easiest to control. After they are mastered she may progress to control faster and larger ones. The direction of the weight shifts also makes a difference. Shifting your weight forward is easiest; shifting it to the side is harder; backwards weight shifts and those that involve turning the trunk are hardest to control whether sitting or standing.

Physical therapists train small weight shifts by working with the children on a mobile surface. For instance, when therapists work with the children sitting or lying on a large ball, the slightest movement will bring about some weight shift. The same is true when the children sit or stand on a rocking board. These activities train children to respond to weight shifts in a general way. In addition, children need to learn to initiate a weight shift and control it in specific situations.

In summary, learning to shift her weight with control enables your child to move independently. Many activities in this book prepare your child for weight shifts or help you to train specific weight shifts you want your child to master.

CLOSED KINETIC CHAIN EXERCISES

One may think of the parts of a leg—the hip, thigh, lower leg, and foot—as a chain. The parts of this chain are linked and move together. The arm is a similar chain. The shoulder, upper arm, lower arm, hand, and fingers are linked and move as a unit. When the end of the chain furthest away from the body is fixed, it is called a closed kinetic (movement) chain.

When you squat down, your feet are not moving but fixed on the floor. When you lie on your stomach and push yourself up with your arms, your hands press against the floor and do not move. Doing squats, pull-ups, or pushups are examples of closed kinetic chain exercises.

In an open kinetic chain, the end furthest away from the body is free. When kicking a ball, your foot moves freely and so does your hand when you reach for something. Kicking, stepping forward, or reaching are examples of open kinetic chain activities.

When doing an open chain activity, your child has to control the direction of the movements around each joint. For instance when throwing a ball, she has to control the direction of the movements around her shoulder, elbow, and wrist joint, as well as open her fingers at the right time so the ball will fly forward. Pressing the ball between her hands—a closed chain activity—is a far simpler movement. The directions of all joint movements are predetermined and the outcome of the movement hardly varies. Doing a movement sequence—pressing the ball, letting go some, and then pressing again—the child's arm muscles are learning to work together in a predictable way.

Physical therapists often use closed kinetic chain exercises when training basic postures and movements. Abnormal reflexes and involuntary movements are less likely to interfere with a closed kinetic chain exercise. Therefore, training of a controlled, coordinated movement pattern becomes possible.

Closed kinetic chain exercises may train skills that require weight shifts and bearing weight with a good posture. These exercises are especially helpful. They train coordinated muscle work, reinforce a good posture, strengthen the muscles, and often stretch important muscles at the same time. The *Sit-Stand-Sit* and *Squat-Stand-Squat* exercises described and illustrated in Chapter 12 are examples of exercises that train good posture and coordinated leg movements as well as stretch and strengthen your child's leg muscles.

The exercise *Rocking on Big Arms* in Chapter 8 is an example of a closed chain arm exercise that combines bearing weight with good posture and shifting weight with control. This exercise shows you how to help your child to push up and then hold the position while you rock her from side to side providing small weight shifts. This strengthens the arm muscles and encourages coordination. At the same time the exercise stretches the muscles that bend the wrist and fingers.

JOINT STABILIZATION

Closed kinetic chain exercises help children in many ways. But in order for the children to play and to walk, physical therapists have to train open chain movements as well. How can this be done? If your child makes abnormal arm movements and cannot reach for a toy, how can she improve? If her legs cross over each time she tries to step, how can she learn to do it better?

Therapists have found that joint stabilization helps to control movement. Joint stabilization means that the therapist holds the joint close to the body and guides the child's movements. For instance, the therapist holds and guides the shoulder joint while the child reaches; or the therapist holds and guides the movement around the hip joint while the child takes a step.

Why is this helpful? When closely observing the children's arm movements, the therapists noted that the abnormal pattern of the arm movement began at the shoulder.

The shoulders moved up and back as the children tried to reach. It gave the movement the wrong start. Therapists found that by helping the children to sit in a good position, relax their shoulders, and stabilizing the shoulder of the reaching arm, they can guide the child's arm to move with a more normal pattern. With consistent training and many repetitions, children slowly learned to reach and touch a toy without assistance.

Joint stabilization during leg movements follows the same principle. The therapist helps the child to stand with a good posture holding onto parallel bars or her walker. The therapist supports the hips, stabilizing the standing leg while guiding the stepping leg. Stepping to the side is practiced similarly. The standing leg is stabilized and the other leg guided to step out to the side.

Skillful and correct joint stabilization is a very helpful tool for therapists. They will use it as needed and fade it out as soon as possible. Regardless of where and how joint stabilization is done, the goal is always for the child to become able to do a useful movement independently without any help.

There are drawbacks to the joint stabilization techniques used by physical therapists. It takes training, skill, and experience to do them. Therefore, they are difficult to teach to parents or other professionals working with the children. If parents master a specific technique helpful with their child they will notice that it is time consuming to implement. It may also be strenuous. For instance, stabilizing your child's hips and guiding her steps is hard work.

Another problem with the technique is that the children may become used to it and rely on it. Instead of becoming independent, they may become dependent on this help from their therapist or parent. Therefore, how to fade out manual joint stabilization has to be as well planned as when to use it.

JOINT STABILIZATION BY POSITIONING

A position may stabilize a joint. In side-lying on the right side, the right shoulder is firmly wedged beneath the body. The left shoulder is stabilized by the effect of gravity. The child's hands rest close to each other. Therapists use side-lying to encourage fine motor skills in a small child who cannot yet control her shoulder muscles and therefore is unable to play lying on her back or tummy. As the therapist places a rattle into one hand, the child may move it, shake it, hold it with both hands, or pass it from one hand to the other. Thereby the child learns to use her hands and gains hand and finger coordination.

GENERAL STABILIZATION TECHNIQUES

These techniques are used to help children with cerebral palsy to "dissociate" or to isolate movements. Dissociating is the term therapists use when describing the ability to move one body part without moving others. If your child moves her head, chest, and arms without moving her hips and legs, she dissociates her upper body from her lower body. If she moves one arm without moving the rest of her body, she is able to dissociate the arm movement.

Your child may be helped to move just one body part by the use of a stabilization technique. The exercise *Kicking with One Leg* in Chapter 12 is an example of how stabilizing helps the child to control the movements of one leg at a time.

Isolating a movement means that the child controls a specific movement such as bending the index finger when she taps a computer key. The therapist may initially stabilize the child's wrist, hand, and other fingers as she learns this discreet movement. Moving one leg to the side without bending the hip or turning the leg is another example of an isolated movement.

Most general stabilization techniques are not difficult. Therapists may teach them to the child's parent or teacher. Specific positions, braces, splints, straps, sandbags, weighted vest, and most recently, even suits, may also be used to provide stabilization to help the child better control her movements.

As with joint stabilization, general stabilization techniques are to be used during initial learning. As soon as possible they are phased out. The goal is for the child to become independent of the help by another person.

There are limits to the benefits of stabilization techniques. They are very helpful when your child needs to learn a new movement but not if she needs to gain control of a position. Let's look at the following situation: You want to teach your child to kick a ball with her right foot. So you support her while she stands on her left foot, ask her to concentrate on her right foot and kick. You make kicking easy and fun and your child succeeds. She learns to swing her leg forward and kick the ball. Now you ask her to kick without you supporting her and she may not be able to do it. The reason is that without your support she cannot stand long enough on her left leg to kick with her right one. Your child learned the movement (kicking) but not the postural control (briefly standing on one leg) to use the movement functionally.

For your child to progress further you had to use exercises or activities, which train postural control and balance. For instance the exercises in Chapter 14 under the heading *Extra Standing Time for the Weaker Leg* would be beneficial. Another possibility would be that you teach your child a self-stabilization technique, which enables her to kick without your help.

SELF-STABILIZATION

Self-stabilization means that children learn to stabilize a joint or their posture by their own action. There are many ways children can stabilize themselves. In the situation mentioned before your child may be encouraged to lean against a wall with her left side when she kicks with her right foot. Or she could hold onto something stable like a doorframe or a banister, brace herself with one hand against a wall, or just touch the wall with one finger to stabilize herself. With no need to support her—she does it herself- you are free to become her partner in the kicking game. With practice your child may slowly become able to support herself less and eventually succeed to kick the ball without holding on.

Usually physical therapists teach self-stabilizing techniques as part of functional skill training. The therapist may ask your child to brace herself with one hand on the bench or on her upper leg as she leans forward to pull up her sock with the other hand. When using the toilet, she may be taught to hold onto a wall bar with one hand while pulling her pants up or down.

When she learns to color or write, the therapist may teach her to hold onto a rod or grab bar with one hand. The bar will be firmly suctioned to her table or desk in such a way that by holding on, her shoulder is pulled slightly forward. This will help her to keep her shoulders in a good position, stabilize her upper body, and make it easier to control the movements of her working hand.

There are many situations in which children may learn to stabilize themselves. It is a useful technique, which is easily adapted to the home or school environment. Therapists may combine joint stabilization they provide with teaching of self-stabilization. This way, as the child's movements improve, the therapist may withdraw her support readily and encourage the child to stabilize herself.

TEACHING FUNCTIONAL SKILLS

How much time should physical therapists spend preparing children for functional skills as opposed to training functional skills directly? For example, should the therapist work on improving a child's sitting balance using a variety of types of therapy equipment? As the child's sitting balance improves, she becomes able to shift her weight with control. This should help her to play or do work while sitting or to move in and out of sitting.

Or should the therapist work with the child as soon as possible on functional skills? In this case, the therapist would spend less time on sitting balance exercises. Instead she would work on functional activities such as doing a specific dressing task while the child sits, or ask the child to move in and out of sitting. The reasoning would be that as the child masters these skills, she would improve her balance and ability to shift her weight with control at the same time.

Which approach will bring better and faster results? There is an ongoing debate and study of this question (Ketelaar, 2001, Ahl Ekstrom, 2005). So far, however, there are no definite answers.

For parents of children with cerebral palsy and similar movement disorders, functional progress is important. You are glad when your child does well with an activity during her therapy session. Yet, when your child becomes able to move in or out of her car seat, you are really happy about it. Your child learned something useful that will make your life easier.

Physical therapy is not just about teaching your child to walk. It is the therapist's goal for your child to become independent with all daily motor tasks. Feel free to ask your therapist to help you with all movement problems your child encounters.

The "Road to Independence" for Children with Cerebral Palsy

"With so much to learn, how will my child ever become independent?" you wonder. Yes, there is much to learn for a child with cerebral palsy or similar movement disorders. But instead of worrying about tomorrow it is best to look at today. Take one day at a time, appreciate small progress, and enjoy major achievements as they are mastered.

The "Road to Independence" lists major achievements you want to look for. Each one will help your child to do more on her own and is a building block for the skills still to be mastered. The initial skills are listed sequentially in the order children usually master them. The first of these may be skipped by children who are able to play with their hands when they lie on their backs or in their infant seats.

Two of the initial skills are listed in bold letters. They are especially important building blocks. Many later skills depend on them. *Holds head and looks around propped on forearms in stomach–lying* is important because it shows that a child has basic head control, has gained some shoulder strength and coordination, and likes to be on her tummy. Your child may master this skill with ease. If not, you want to provide as much help as needed. Your special attention and training will make a difference. Chapter 6 and 8 address this in more detail.

"Bunny" – from stomach-lying: child pulls both legs up and props on both arms is another early skill printed with bold letters. Moving into the "bunny" position is the easiest way children with cerebral palsy and similar movement disorders can lift their body off the surface. The sooner your child learns this, the better. As she becomes independent with this skill and does it many times during the day, the strength and coordination of her trunk, shoulder, and arm muscles will improve. At the same time, she will be challenged to shift her weight and keep her balance in ways not possible if she just played lying on the floor.

The intermediate skills are clustered. The order they are mastered may vary from child to child. *Sits and stands holding onto a bar* is listed in the beginning to assure that it is trained early. Chapter 12 explains the reasoning for this. The sitting and kneeling skills are listed side by side. It is good to work on them concurrently. Children with hypotonia may show steady progress with floor sitting. Children with hypertonia often have difficulty there. (See Chapter 10 for details.) They may show better progress with kneeling. Training sitting and variations of kneeling concurrently will assure that the children progress to the best of their ability. Training kneeling after a child is able to sit could delay her progress.

Training of pulling to stand, cruising along furniture, and assisted stair walking are listed with walking with an assistive device. Again, these skills are best trained concurrently. They improve your child's leg muscle strength and coordination. (See Chapter 12 for details.)

The advanced skills start with *Stands without Support,* which is printed in bold letters. Gaining independent standing balance is the key to all advanced skills. After your child learns to stand without holding on, training of walking without arm support becomes a possibility.

The "Road to Independence" is meant to be a general guideline of how children with cerebral palsy or similar movement disorders master gross motor skills. It does not tell or predict the order in which your child may learn the skills. Your child's gross motor development will depend on her specific potentials and problems.

"ROAD TO INDEPENDENCE" SKILLS GUIDELINE

INITIAL SKILLS:

- Brings hands together and plays in side-lying. *(photo 4.1)*
- Holds head in the middle, brings hands together, and plays in an infant seat. *(photo 4.2)*
- **Holds head and looks around propped on forearms in stomach-lying.** *(photo 4.3)*
- Lifts feet off the floor in back-lying and rolls over. *(photo 4.4)*
- Plays and moves about on stomach. *(photo 4.5)*
- Sits with both arms propped. *(photo 4.6)*
- **"Bunny" from stomach-lying: child pulls both legs up and props on both arms.** *(photo 4.7)*

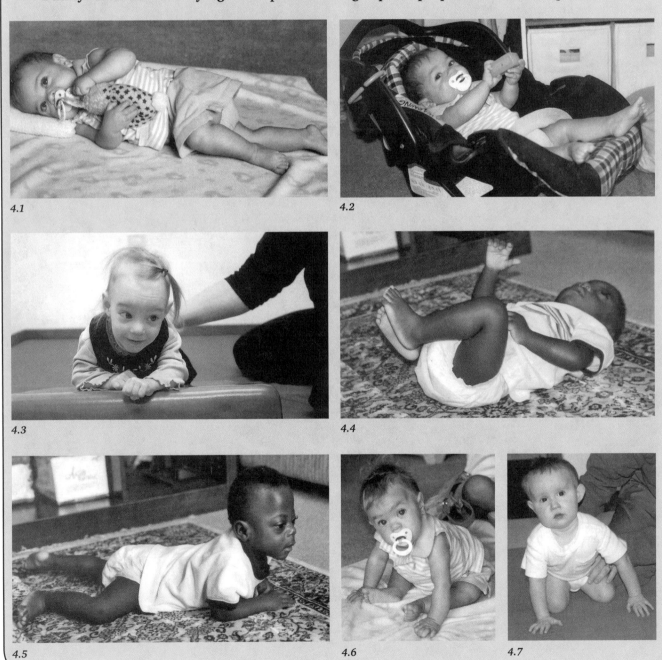

4.1

4.2

4.3

4.4

4.5

4.6

4.7

(Continued on next page.)

(Continued from previous page.)

INTERMEDIATE SKILLS I:

- Sits and stands holding onto a bar. *(photo 4.8a & 4.8b)*
- Pulls from bunny position to kneeling at a box and plays. *(photo 4.9)*
- Sits with some arm support and plays. *(photo 4.10)*
- Plays in bunny position. *(photo 4.11)*
- Plays in heel sitting and moves in/out of position. *(photo 4.12)*
- Sits without arm support and moves in/out of sitting. *(photo 4.13)*

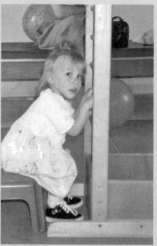
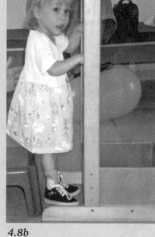

4.8a
4.8b

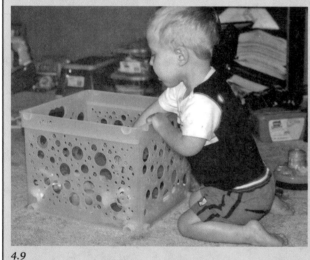

4.9

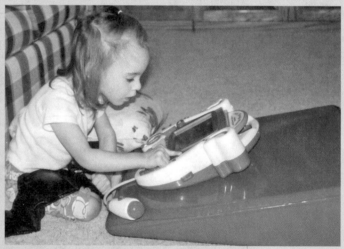

4.10

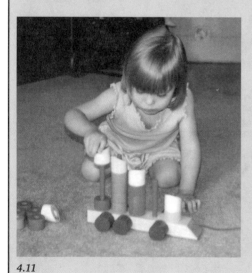

4.11

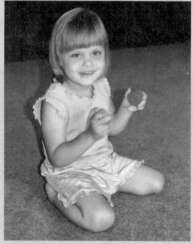

4.12

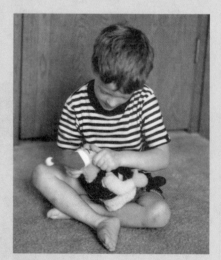

4.13

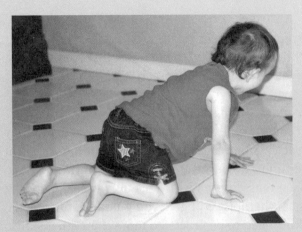

4.14

INTERMEDIATE SKILLS II:

- Crawls on hands and knees. *(photo 4.14)*
- Sits well on a bench or chair. *(photo 4.15)*
- Pulls to stand at furniture, plays, and cruises. *(photo 4.16)*
- Walks with a walker. *(photo 4.17)*
- Walks with forearm crutches. *(photo 4.18)*
- Walks stairs with assistance.

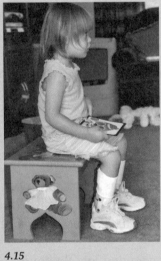

4.15

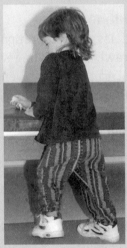

4.16

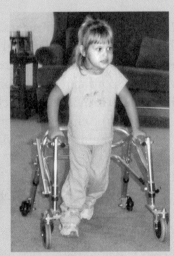

4.17

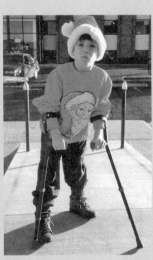

4.18

ADVANCED SKILLS:

- **Stands without Support.** *(photo 4.19)*
- Walks without support. *(photo 4.20)*
- Walks up and down stairs, walks up and down curbs, and may run.

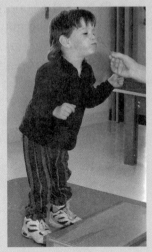

4.19

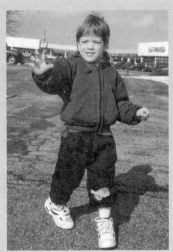

4.20

Frequently Asked Questions

Q. *"How long will it take our son Hayden to learn each skill?"*
A. This varies greatly from child to child. Hayden may learn a few skills rather quickly, while others may require weeks or even months of daily practice.

Q. *"Should we work with Hayden on one skill at a time?"*
A. In general, it is good to work on several skills at a time. As mentioned you may want to work on sitting and kneeling at the same time and practice standing with arm support also on the same day. Some times, however, it helps to concentrate on one skill and practice it over and over (see massed practice). This all varies depending on circumstances. Your child's physical therapist will give you guidance for specific situations. She will explain which skills need to be practiced more than other skills.

Q. *"Does Celeste have to crawl in order to walk?"*
A. Children with developmental delays or cerebral palsy may learn to walk with a walker without first being able to crawl. Yet, crawling will help Celeste in many ways. It teaches her coordinated reciprocal arm and leg movements and strengthens her hip, shoulder, and arm muscles. Few children walk independently without ever crawling. An exception is the child with hemiplegia whose arm is seriously affected by cerebral palsy. She will be unable to crawl, but still progress to independent walking.

Q. *"Does Celeste have to walk with a walker before she walks on her own?"*
A. No. Not all children with cerebral palsy walk with a walker first, but many do.

Q. *"Our son Mohsen has hemiplegia. Only one side of his body is affected by cerebral palsy. How will he develop gross motor skills?"*
A. On his own, Mohsen will rely mostly on his stronger arm and leg. By doing so, he may learn most skills almost as quickly as children without cerebral palsy until it is time to walk. Now the abnormal muscle tone, the lack of coordination, and the weakness of the affected leg may delay the onset of walking. Nevertheless, he will progress to independent walking.

It is best for Mohsen to receive physical therapy early. It will assure that he uses his affected arm and leg as much as possible and does not "neglect" them. Even though it is not essential that children with hemiplegia crawl, they benefit a great deal from crawling. The more Mohsen crawls, the stronger and more coordinated his affected arm and leg become. For the rest of his life, he will benefit from crawling.

5

Flexible Muscles and Joints

If your child has been diagnosed with cerebral palsy, you were probably told that his developmental delay was caused by damage to the nervous system. The brain was sending the wrong messages to the muscles and this caused the muscles not to work correctly. Your baby's joints and bones were just as perfect as any other baby's. Although this is true, older children with cerebral palsy may develop problems with joints and bones, which may be just as worrisome to parents as the delays their child may be experiencing in achieving important gross motor skills.

Possible Muscle Problems

"If my baby was born with good joints and bones, why does this change when he gets older?" you wonder. It has to do with the way muscles and bones grow. Bones have growth plates and they grow as children age. Muscles, on the other hand, grow longer when they are stretched. *As the bones grow and children move, the muscles are stretched, causing them to grow.* This way the length of the muscles will match the length of the bones. This is how it should be—muscles of the right length work best.

Let us use the growth of the biceps muscle as an example. The biceps is the muscle of the upper arm that bulges out when the elbow bends. One end of the biceps attaches to the shoulder and the upper arm bone (humerus) and the other end attaches to a lower arm bone (radius). When the elbow is straightened, the biceps is stretched. As the arm bones grow, the biceps is stretched more each time the elbow is straightened. This stretch causes the biceps to grow.

When the arm bones of a child with cerebral palsy grow, however, the biceps may not match the growth of the bones. This happens if the child cannot fully straighten his elbow on his own due to spasticity of the muscles that bend the elbow, lack of strength and control of the muscles that straighten the elbow, abnormal reflexes, or a combination of all three. Consequently, the biceps muscle is never stretched to its full length. The normal stretch with the message from the bones: "Hello, we are growing, hurry and catch up!" never occurs. Therefore, the biceps does not grow even though the arm bones are getting longer. At the same time, the triceps muscle opposite of the biceps on the back of the upper arm is constantly stretched over the bent elbow. Consequently, this muscle becomes longer than necessary.

Cerebral palsy, then, is the secondary reason that the muscles fail to grow appropriately. The primary cause is the lack of full joint motion. Cerebral palsy is the reason that your one-year-old cannot straighten his elbows, but you can straighten them for him. And if you do so each day, the biceps muscles will be helped to grow, as they should. ***Daily stretching will help prevent muscle shortening***.

The benefits of preventing the muscles from becoming too short are enormous. Muscles of the right length work best. They are stronger than muscles that are either too short or too long. Muscles of the right length are easier for your child to use and therefore make learning new skills easier. ***A short muscle is not only less useful, it interferes with skill acquisition and the daily care*** of children with cerebral palsy. If the biceps become so short that the elbows can no longer be straightened, it will interfere with weight bearing on arms and learning essential skills such as catching yourself with outstretched arms or crawling. Additionally, the bent arms will make dressing the child difficult.

The biceps of the upper arms, the hamstrings at the back of the thighs, the inner thigh muscles, and the calf muscles are most likely to shorten as the result of insufficient use. They are big, strong muscles which work on two joints. The biceps, for instance, not only bend the elbows, they also help lift the arms at the shoulder joints. The hamstrings bend the knees and help to straighten the hips. The inner thigh muscles pull the legs together and also help bend the knees. The calf muscles push the feet down and also help bend the knees.

Short inner thigh muscles will interfere with floor sitting or daily care. Short calf muscles limit how much the ankle joints bend and thus may prevent the heels from touching the floor in standing. Short hamstring muscles will limit the length of each forward step or even hinder the knees from being straightened. Short hamstrings also interfere with floor sitting. Their pull tips the hip bone (pelvis) backwards and makes you sit with a rounded low back. These muscles play a major role in the way your child sits, stands, or walks.

Possible Joint Problems

CONTRACTURES

When a joint is not straightened for weeks or months, the fibrous tissues (ligaments) around the joint that hold the joint together are affected. Some become shorter and some longer. These changes will limit the range of motion of the joint. Now it is not only the short muscles, but also the short ligaments, which prevent the full joint motion. ***This is called joint contracture.*** A joint contracture that persists will, over time, bring about changes to the bones at the joint and ultimately become irreversible. Stretching at this point will not reverse the contracture.

Understanding how a joint contracture develops will help to prevent it. Let's use the knee joint as an ex-

> ## WHAT IS RANGE OF MOTION?
>
> **Range of Motion (ROM)** is the natural distance and direction a joint moves.
>
> **Active Range of Motion (AROM)** is how far the muscles affecting the joint can move the joint. That is, it refers to how far the person himself can move the joint.
>
> **Passive Range of Motion (PROM)** is how far a joint can be moved passively. That is, it refers to how far someone else can move the person's joint.

ample. Several two-joint muscles affect the knee joint, including the muscles of the back of the thigh—the hamstrings. The hamstring muscles are stretched to their full length (full range of motion) when the knee is straight and the leg is 70 to 85 degrees bent at the hip. If a child is unable to get his leg into this position, a knee flexion contracture can develop. This means the knee can no longer be fully straightened. The development of knee flexion contractures can be categorized into three stages:

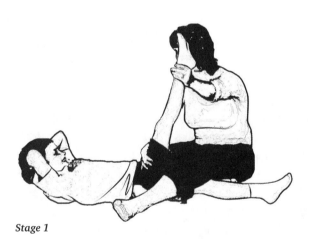

Stage 1

Stage 1: Little or no active range of motion with full passive range of motion. Due to weakness, spasticity, or lack of coordination, the child is unable to straighten his knee and move his straight leg forward. Another person can straighten the child's knee and move the leg through its full range of motion.

Daily stretching exercises can be done with ease and will help to assure that full passive range of the hamstrings is maintained as the child matures and his bones grow longer.

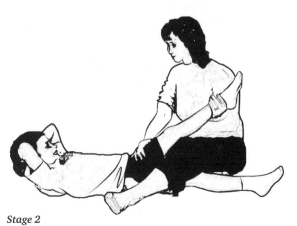

Stage 2

Stage 2: Little or no active range of motion with limited passive range of motion. The child is unable to straighten his knee and move his straight leg forward. Another person can straighten the child's knee fully, but the straight leg can no longer be moved into 70 degree of hip flexion. When the child lies on his back and the straight leg is lifted up (bent at the hip) the knee soon begins to bend. How soon the knee will bend depends on how tight the hamstrings have become.

At this point, stretching exercises have to be done with care. Daily stretching will prevent the muscles from shortening further. Over time the daily stretching routine may improve the flexibility of the hamstrings and full passive range of motion may be regained.

Stage 3: No active range of motion and significantly reduced or no passive joint range. The child is not able to straighten the knee on his own and another person cannot straighten the knee either. This is called a knee flexion contracture.

It is very difficult to loosen a joint contracture with stretching exercises. The longer the contracture persists the less likely it is that it can be reversed.

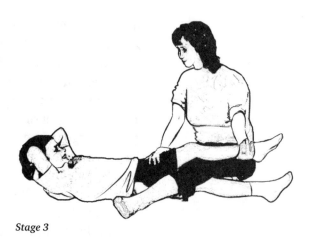

Stage 3

JOINT SUBLUXATION OR DISLOCATION

Another serious consequence of short muscles is that they place stress on the joints. *The constant pull of tight, short muscles will affect how joints grow.* Short biceps will affect the elbow joints. Short hamstring and inner thigh muscles will affect the hip joints. The bones will grow in such a way that joint subluxations or dislocations become more likely. (A subluxation means that the joint has moved partially out of its socket; a dislocation means that the joint has moved completely out of its socket.)

Daily Stretching to Prevent Muscle and Joint Problems

You can prevent your child's muscles from becoming too short. Daily stretching a muscle will help to maintain its length. Stretching is easily done when your child is small. His joints and ligaments are soft and his muscles flexible. Most babies like to be touched. They usually enjoy range of motion exercises and don't mind stretching.

The problem is that you have to do stretches every day. While your child is small, you need to spend so much time feeding, dressing, and cleaning him that the additional time needed to fully straighten his joints is insignificant and is easily fit into the daily routine. Continuing to do daily stretches with an older, independent, or opinionated child is another matter. For children, the stretches become boring, and may be somewhat uncomfortable. For parents, doing the stretches becomes more strenuous as the child's limbs grow longer and heavier. Sometimes it just seems easier to skip the stretching exercises. Unfortunately, this will have its consequences. A couple of weeks without any stretches is enough for some muscles to lose the length achieved by previous stretching. The next time the muscle is stretched, it will be more uncomfortable and the child will like it even less.

A parent may decide: "This is too difficult for me. I'd better let the therapist do the stretches." And it is true that physical therapists do the needed stretches as part of each therapy session. The problem is that therapy sessions are usually once per week, and this is not enough.

The shorter a muscle becomes, the more difficult it is to stretch. There comes a point when manual stretching loses its effectiveness. Perhaps weeks of serial casting may now be the only way to lengthen the muscle. (Chapter 17 has information concerning serial casting.) Surgery can also be used for this purpose. But surgery will not lengthen the muscle fibers. It will increase the length of the tendon the muscle is wrapped in. A surgically lengthened muscle tends to become weaker.

In summary, it is very important that your child's muscles match the length of the bones they are paired with. You want to keep them this way. Daily stretching will help do this.

How to Do Stretching Exercises

Like many parents, you may be familiar with stretching exercises. You may have done them when you trained for a sport or you may stretch when you do a regular exercise routine. This knowledge and experience is very helpful when you do stretching exercises with your child. There are, however, special considerations and precautions when stretching a child with cerebral palsy. Your child's therapist will explain them to you, decide which stretches your child needs, and demonstrate them.

Technique is important when you do stretching exercises. The joint needs to be well stabilized. Furthermore, if an exercise calls for straightening or bending, no twisting or turning may accompany the motion. Parents are advised **not to attempt** stretching exercises on their own. Instead, practice them with the therapist's guidance before you work with your child at home.

Be forewarned that it may take several days or more than a week before you and your child are comfortable with the daily stretching routine. For reassurance that you are doing the stretches correctly, it is a good idea to have the therapist watch you doing them at the next visit.

The following are general guidelines for stretching a child with cerebral palsy:

- **Move slowly.** As explained in Chapter 3, if you stretch a spastic muscle slowly, the same resistance is felt until the muscle is stretched to its full length. If you do it quickly the resistance increases and stops the movement before the muscle has reached its full length.

- **Position your child well.** Closely follow the therapist's instructions. Stretching may be easiest to do when your child rests on his back. But this is the position in which abnormal reflexes are more likely to occur. Therefore, you need to take precautions to minimize these reflexes, as your therapist advises, or an alternative position may have to be used.

- **Talk to your child.** Have a conversation with your child when you do stretches. Talking connects you and keeps you in tune with your child. If your child loves music, sing a song to him. The sound of your voice makes your child comfortable and puts him at ease, and the conversation will distract him. The more relaxed your child is, the more effective the stretch is. You want to create a calm atmosphere. Remember, spasticity increases with excitement, discomfort, or any other emotional response. Nothing is accomplished if your child fights you and pushes against you.

- **Know when to stop and hold the stretch.** When you stretch yourself, you can feel when a muscle has reached its full length. Further stretching becomes uncomfortable and then painful. When you stretch your child, it is important to carefully watch his face for any signs of discomfort. If this happens, immediately stop stretching the muscle and reduce your pressure. *Do not think that you can judge by the resistance you feel when to stop stretching.* Small children have soft joints and ligaments and their muscles are weak. If your child is relaxed or has low muscle tone, it is easy to stretch too much. This could seriously damage his muscles and joints.

- **Do not overstretch a muscle.** This is advice for parents who have been following a regular stretching routine with their child. After weeks of regular stretching, there will come a time when, for instance, the hamstring muscles achieved a normal length and show good flexibility. At this point, you are advised to bring the leg up to the highest position without stretching it any further. Normal flexibility is good and nothing is gained by too much flexibility. Maintaining normal flexibility as your child grows is the goal of the regular stretching routine.

The following are examples of stretching exercises. *Only use them as your child's therapist directs you.* The therapist knows your child and will be able to make any special adjustments that may be needed.

ARM STRETCHES

Arm Stretches in Back-Lying

Your child lies on his back. You kneel facing him. Place your left thumb or index finger into his left palm and between his left thumb and index finger. Drape your other fingers around his hand and wrist. With your right hand, grasp your child's left shoulder and upper arm and gently move the arm over your child's chest toward the opposite shoulder as far as it will go with ease. Then:

1. Gently move the left hand as far as the therapist recommends or until the elbow is straight. The shoulder should not lift off the surface. Hold the stretch for 30 seconds while you talk to your child (photo 5.1).
2. Move the straight arm forward (photo 5.2) and upward as far as the therapist recommends or until it touches the floor beside your child's head (photo 5.3). Hold the stretch for 30 seconds while you talk to your child.

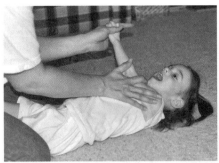

5.1

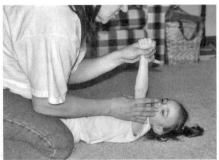

5.2

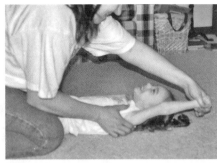

5.3

3. Move the straight arm forward and then out to the side as far as the therapist recommends or until it touches the floor (photo 5.4). Hold the stretch for 30 seconds while you talk to your child.
4. Move the straight arm forward and then slant it diagonally across your child's body until the palm of his hand touches his right thigh (photo 5.5). Hold the stretch for 30 seconds while you talk to your child.
5. Move the slanted arm straight up and out to the side until the back of the hand rests on the floor with the palm facing upward (photo 5.6). Hold the stretch for 30 seconds while you talk to your child.
6. Reverse the position of your hands and stretch your child's right arm.

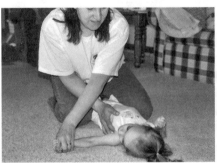

5.4

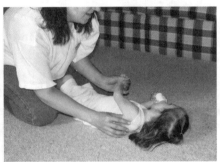

5.5

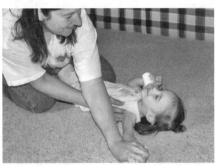

5.6

Note: All arm movements begin at the shoulder joint. Your hand at the upper arm will start the movements. Your other hand follows the movement, supporting your child's lower arm and hand. Do not pull at your child's hand.

Arm Stretch in Sitting

This exercise and the following exercises show the same stretches done in a sitting position, which may be more pleasant and comfortable for you and your child. This way, however, you cannot observe your child's face. Use this position after you have determined your child's level of tolerance and according to the directions of your child's therapist.

Your child sits on your lap with his back against your trunk. Place your left thumb or index finger into his right palm and between his right thumb and index finger. Drape your other fingers around his hand and wrist. Grasp his right shoulder and upper arm with your right hand.

1. Gently move the arm over the chest as far as it will go with ease (photo 5.7). Now straighten the elbow fully or as much as the therapist recommends. Hold the stretch for 30 seconds while you talk to your child.

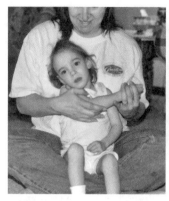

5.7

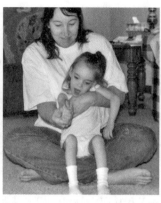

5.8

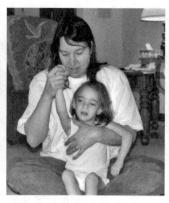

5.9

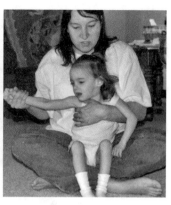

5.10

2. Change your hand position and hold his right hand with your right hand. Move the straight right arm forward (photo 5.8) and then up as far as the therapist recommends or until it touches your child's right ear (photo 5.9). Hold the stretch for 30 seconds while you talk to your child.

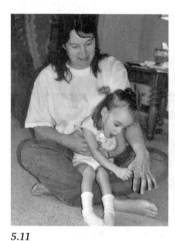

5.11

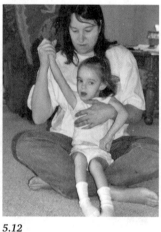

5.12

3. Move the straight arm forward and then out to the side as far as the therapist recommends (photo 5.10). Hold the stretch for 30 seconds while you talk to your child.

4. Move the straight arm forward and then slant it diagonally across your child's body until the palm of his hand touches his left leg or crosses over it (photo 5.11). Hold the stretch for 30 seconds while you talk to your child.

5. Move the slanted arm straight up and out to the side as far as the therapist recommends (photo 5.12). Hold the stretch for 30 seconds while you talk to your child.

6. Reverse the position of your hands and stretch your child's left arm.

Forearm, Wrist, and Hand Stretches

Your child sits on your lap with his back against you. With your right hand on his right shoulder and upper arm, move his arm forward and over so you can comfortably hold his right hand with your left hand and stabilize your child's wrist. The wrist should be straight, not bent forward or backwards, with the thumb pointing up.

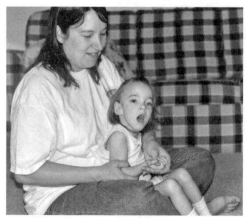

5.13

1. Slowly rotate the wrist as far as the therapist recommends or until the palm is facing up (photo 5.13). Slowly straighten the elbow as much as possible (photo 5.14). Hold the stretch for 30 seconds while you talk to your child. Return your child's hand to the starting position with the thumb pointing up.

2. Your right hand supports your child's right elbow and lower arm. With your left hand, slowly bend the wrist slightly toward the thumb side, as shown in the illustration (illustration 5.14a). This is a small movement. Hold the stretch for 30 seconds while you talk to your child.

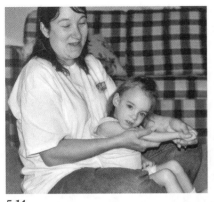

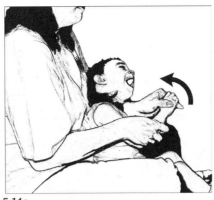

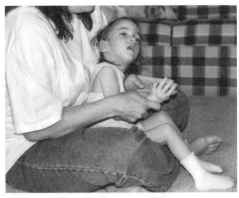

5.14   5.14a   5.15

3. Slowly bend your child's open hand backwards. The movement is from the wrist. Your mild pressure is against his palm. After you move the wrist as far as the therapist recommends, gently straighten his fingers (photo 5.15). Hold the stretch for 30 seconds while you talk to your child.
4. Reverse the position of your hands and stretch your child's left wrist and hand.

Finger and Thumb Wiggles

Hold your child's hand in a position that is comfortable for both of you, with your child's elbow bent and your hand stabilizing his wrist. Start with the little finger.

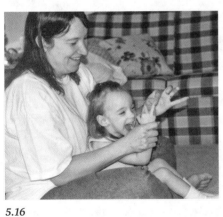

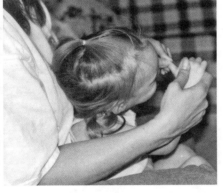

Gently straighten each finger and, with a slight pull, circle it around 5 times clockwise and 5 times counterclockwise (photo 5.16). Do the same with the thumb.

Next hold your child's thumb and gently spread it away from his fingers out to the side and hold the stretch for 30 seconds (photo 5.17).

Repeat the stretches with the fingers and thumb of your child's other hand.

5.16   5.17

LEG STRETCHES

One Leg Up – One Leg Down (Hamstrings Stretch)

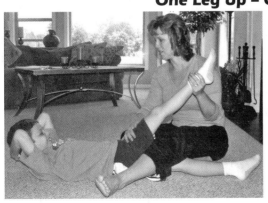

Your child lies on his back. You sit at his left side near his lower legs, facing him. Lift his left leg and slide your leg under his left and over his right leg. This way you are pinning his straight right leg down to the floor. Now, raise his left leg, with knee straight, up as high as it will go (photo 5.18). Hold the stretch for 1 minute while you talk to your child.

Do the same stretch holding the left leg down and lifting the right leg up.

5.18

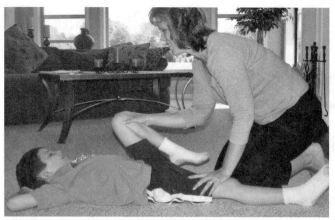

5.19

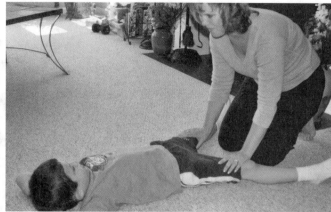

5.20

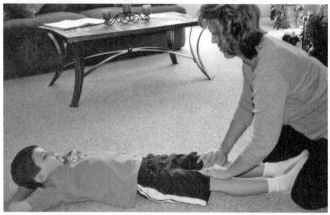

5.21

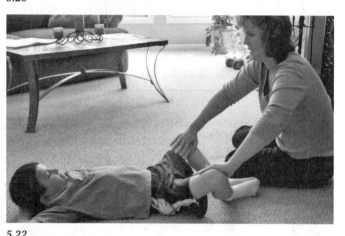

5.22

One Knee Up—One Leg Down (Hip Stretch)

Your child lies on his back. You kneel facing him. Bend both knees and move them up toward his tummy. Next hold the left leg where it is while you straighten and lower the right leg to the floor (photo 5.19). Hold the stretch for 1 minute while you talk to your child.

Do the same stretch holding the right knee up and the left leg down.

Windshield Wiper Stretch (Inner Thigh Muscle Stretch)

Your child lies on his back with his legs straight and toes pointing up or slightly out. Grasp his legs above his knees and spread your child's legs apart as far as they will go (photo 5.20). Hold the stretch for 1 minute while you talk to your child.

Rolling Out Stretch (Hip Rotator Muscle Stretch)

Your child lies on his back with his legs straight. Grasp his legs above his knees and roll your child's legs out as far as they will go (photo 5.21). Hold the stretch for 1 minute while you talk with your child.

Butterfly Stretch (Rotator and Inner Thigh Muscles Stretch)

Your child lies on his back (photo 5.22) or sits on the floor (photo 5.23) with his legs straight in front of him. Bend both knees and gently push them out to the sides as far as they will go. Hold the stretch for 1 minute while you talk with your child.

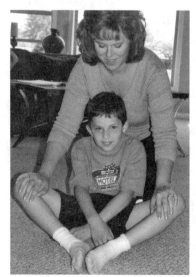

5.23

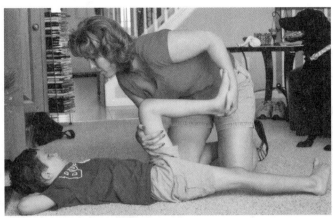

5.24

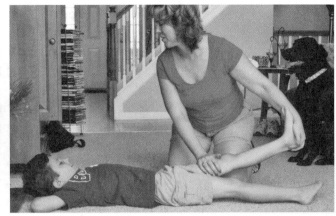

5.25

Calf Muscle Stretch

Your child lies on his back or sits on your lap with his back against you. With his right knee bent, cup your hand around his heel and gently pull the heel down and push the foot up as far as it will go (photo 5.24). Pause, making sure the foot is in a good position, facing forward, and not pointing inward or outward. With the foot in this position, gently straighten the knee (photo 5.25). Hold the stretch for 1 minute while you talk to your child.

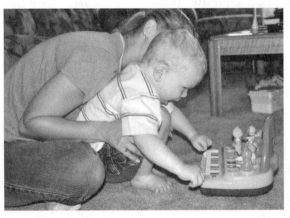

5.26

Calf Muscle Stretch in Deep Squatting

Place your child's favorite toy on the floor. With his feet shoulder-width apart and toes pointing forward or slightly outward, help him to squat down in front of it while keeping his feet flat on the floor. Help him to maintain the position by placing your hands over his knees. Encourage your child to lean forward, relax, and play for a few minutes (photo 5.26).

Note: Play in squatting is a very effective way to stretch the calf muscles, which attach just below the knee. Once they become used to this position, children tolerate it very well. Ankle stretches in back-lying are usually less well tolerated. Yet, they stretch the other calf muscles, which cross the knee joint. These muscles will not be stretched in squatting. Your therapist may recommend that you routinely do both stretches with your child.

Ankle Rolls

Your child lies on his back or sits in your lap. Hold his right leg still with one hand and grasp his right foot with the other. Gently circle it, five times clockwise and then five times counterclockwise. Repeat the exercise with his left foot (photo 5.27).

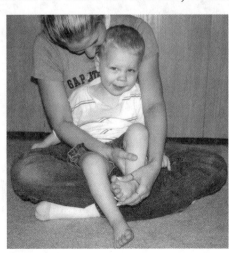

5.27

Wiggle Each Toe

Grasp your child's toes one at a time and gently stretch and move them around (photo 5.28). Play "This Little Piggy Went to Market."

Note: Relax and keep it light. These stretches should not be strenuous for you or your child and should not be painful. ***The key is to do them regularly.***

As you gently hold your child's leg or arm in a stretching position, you may notice that after 15 to 30 seconds the leg or arm will stretch a little further. This lets you know that your child is getting a good relaxing stretch and that his range of motion is increasing.

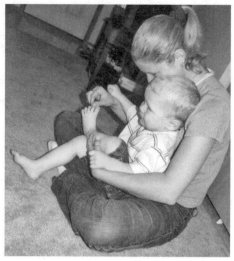

5.28

Stretching Exercises for the Older Child

As your child grows older, he may become able to do stretching exercises on his own. Self-stretching will make him more independent and responsible. It will build the foundation for a lifetime habit of taking good care of himself.

Initially, you want to be next to your child as he does his stretches. Later, after you are assured that he does a good job on his own, you may reduce your supervision.

Stretching the Leg in Sitting (Hamstrings Stretch)

Your child sits in a chair or in his wheelchair in front of a low table or another chair. Helping with his hands as much as needed, he places his right leg with toes pointing up onto the table. Now he relaxes—leans backwards—and fully straightens the right knee (photo 5.29). Keeping the knee straight, he then sits up as straight as possible, leaning forward from the hip—with arm support if needed— and holds the position for 1 minute (photo 5.30). He will feel the stretch behind his right knee and below his right buttock. Next he repeats the stretch with the left leg.

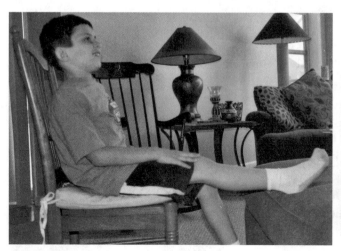

5.29

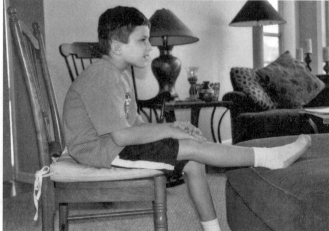

5.30

Variation: To stretch the hamstrings more, your child does the following: After he sits straight with his right leg stretched out, he leans forward from the hip, bringing his tummy closer to his thigh. He will feel the stretch behind his right knee and below his right buttock. Ask him to hold the stretch for 1 minute.

Next he does the same stretch with the left leg.

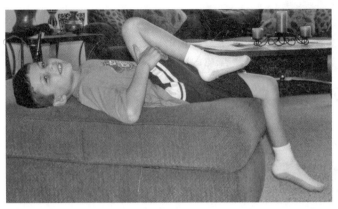

5.31

One Knee Up—One Leg Down Stretch (Hip Flexor Stretch)

Your child sits at the edge of his bed or another similar surface. He pulls the right knee up towards his chest and rolls backwards into back-lying with the left leg hanging over the edge of the bed. Ask him to relax and slowly pull the right leg closer towards his chest until he feels a stretch in front of the left hip (photo 5.31). He holds the position for 1 minute.

Next he repeats the stretch with the left knee.

Leaning Forward Stretch (Inner Thigh and Buttock Muscles Stretch)

Your child sits at the edge of a chair with his legs as far apart as possible and feet flat on the floor. Ask him to sit up straight. Then, bending from the hip, lean far forward until he feels a stretch in his inner thighs and his buttocks (photo 5.32). He holds the stretch for 1 minute.

Note: Your child should not feel a stretch in his low back. If he does, tell him to keep his trunk straight as he leans forward. Allow him to brace himself with his arms as he holds the stretch.

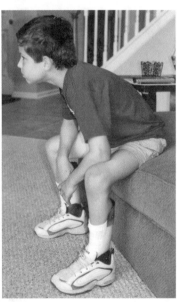

5.32

Inner Thigh Muscle Stretch In Sitting

Your child sits on a sofa, bed, or similar furniture. He pulls the right knee up—with the help of his hands if needed. He places the right foot next to the left thigh. He sits straight up, leans slightly forward, and pushes the right knee down with his right hand (photo 5.33). He will feel the stretch in his inner thigh muscles. He holds the stretch for 1 minute.

He repeats the stretch with the left leg.

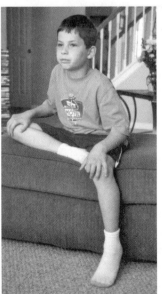

5.33

Calf Muscle Stretch in Standing

Your child stands facing a wall with his left leg forward in front of his right leg. His toes point straight ahead, not turned in or out. With his hands, he braces himself against the wall. He bends his left knee and keeps his right knee straight. Tell him to lean forward until he feels a stretch in his right calf muscles (photo 5.34). Ask

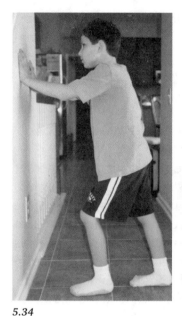

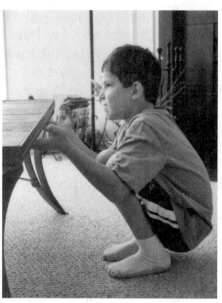

5.34   5.35

him to hold the position for 1 minute. The heel of the right foot should not come up off the floor.

He repeats the stretch with his right leg in front of his left leg.

Calf Muscle Stretch in Squatting

Your child stands in front of a heavy piece of furniture, supports himself with his arms at the furniture, and bends his knees and hips while keeping his feet flat on the floor and toes pointing forward or slightly outward (photo 5.35). Ask him to hold the lowest possible position for 1 minute.

Frequently Asked Questions

Q. *"Should I do all these exercises with my child?"*
A. This is a question for your child's therapist to answer. These range of motion exercises and stretches are a substitute for movements your child is not able to do on his own. As your child improves and his active range of movement increases, some of the stretches will no longer be necessary.

For instance, when your child starts to crawl on hands and knees, he most likely has gained control of his arm movements. The shoulder, elbow, wrist, and even finger and thumb joints will stay flexible and the muscles will not shorten. The range of motion and stretching exercises for the arms are not needed anymore. Remember, though: All rules have exceptions and your child's therapist will have the final say.

Q. *"Which of the leg stretches are most important?"*
A. The hamstring stretch, the hip stretches, and the calf muscles stretch are most important. Most children with cerebral palsy need them throughout childhood. These daily stretches will help keep the leg muscles at a good length and prevent the serious medical problems due to muscle tightness.

Q. *"If these stretches are so important, when should I start doing them with my child?"*
A. It is best to start doing them when your child is still an infant. Instead of waiting until your child needs them—translated: "Oh, no, his muscles are getting tight"—start them when they are easy to do. This way, stretching will not be uncomfortable for your child, you will learn the stretching techniques well, your child will get used to them, and, best of all, you will establish a daily habit and a special time for you both.

Q. *"My daughter, Christie, does not yet crawl or walk. Should I do all the leg stretches with her?"*
A. Not all children benefit from the windshield wiper, rolling out, or butterfly stretch. *Do not do them unless Christie's therapist tells you to.*

Q. *"My daughter, Amanda, does not like her arms stretched. She immediately pulls her arms away and fights me. I try to be very gentle, but nothing helps. What should I do?"*
A. Talk to Amanda's therapist about it. He or she will give you the most knowledgeable advice.

As a person who does not know you or Amanda, I recommend that you observe Amanda and find out how much and how far she moves her arms on her own. For instance, how far does she straighten her elbows when she plays and reaches for something? During the daily stretching time, move her arm this much, no more, and hold it while you talk to Amanda. Do this for a week or until she relaxes with you. Then, very gradually, straighten her elbow a little more than she would on her own. If she does not resist, you are on the right track.

Q. *"Does it help to do the stretching after Amanda takes her bath at night?"*
A. Yes. It is a good routine to do the stretches after a warm bath. Even then it is important to do them gently and be mindful of your child's reaction.

Q. *"Will rubbing the inside of Amanda's elbow help?"*
A. Yes, rubbing the muscle that you are stretching may help. But do not stretch the muscle forcefully and then rub it to make it tolerable. ***Never use force.***

Q. *"My son, John, tolerates it well when my wife stretches him but complains when I do it. What am I doing wrong?"*
A. Have John's therapist observe as you do the stretches and follow his or her advice. Men are physically stronger than women. Therefore, your stretch could be more forceful (and more painful) than you believe.

Q. *"How long will it take my child to get used to stretching?"*
A. This varies from child to child. Whenever your child complains, reduce your pressure and give only a very mild stretch. If your child continues to complain for three days in a row, stop the daily routine until you have a chance to talk to his therapist.

Q. *"Do stretches have to be done as shown here?"*
A. No, there are many ways to stretch muscles. These stretching and range of motion exercises are examples of how to stretch particular muscles. Other ways may work better for your child. It is always best to follow your therapist's instructions.

Q. *"Our son, Jordan, always had good flexibility. Yet, his physician tells us now that his hip-bones are coming out of their sockets and he may need surgery. Why is this happening?"*
A. Unfortunately, in spite of good flexibility, some children with cerebral palsy do develop hip problems. Imbalance of muscle strength, strong abnormal reflexes, or abnormal postures may be some of the contributing factors.

Q. *"Why should I hold the stretches for 30 seconds or for 1 minute?"*
A. Research has shown that hamstring stretches done by an average adult are most effective if done for 30 seconds once a day. A stretch shorter than 30 seconds is not as effective. Longer or repeated stretching does not increase the effectiveness (Bandy, 1997 and 1998).

A recent study of children six years of age and older with cerebral palsy showed good results with one-minute long hamstring stretches repeated five times (Stuberg, 2005). However, no study has been done to find out if one stretch a day would be as good as five stretches. Until more research can be done, one daily stretch seems to do the job instead of five repetitions, which can be very time consuming.

The recommendation for stretching the arms is 30 seconds because the arm muscles are easier to stretch than the leg muscles and 30 seconds seems to be sufficient.

6

Head-Up

"Yes, Keith is able to hold his head up well," confirms the physical therapist. You had been waiting for a response, wondering why the therapist had been talking and smiling at your seven-month-old baby while holding him up in the air this way and that way. Wasn't the physical therapist supposed to look at Keith's muscles? Nothing like this had happened. She just had played with Keith and was having fun, it seemed. "Keith has very good head control," the therapist repeats. You are happy about the good news, but you are unsure what it means.

Head control is a crucial developmental milestone. It is typically mastered in infancy, before children sit, crawl, stand, or walk. Without head control, children will not acquire any of these advanced skills.

There are two aspects of head control. One is the ability to move your head and the other is the ability to hold it still and to automatically adjust the head position as you move about. This is a very important function. To focus your eyes on objects or to eat, you must be able to hold your head still. When the therapist played with Keith, she had been testing his ability to hold his head in various positions.

The Importance of Head Control

You have head control. You can hold your head up, you can turn it, you can tilt it, and you can hold your head in numerous different positions. Best of all, you can hold your head still with your eyes level even when your body twists, bends, or turns. These abilities come naturally to you. While you drive, you reach inside the glove compartment and get your sunglasses out while keeping your eyes on the road and your head upright and still. You can kick off those pinching shoes, but your head remains still. If the sun beats in through the car windows and you get too warm, you can even take off your sweater without moving your head while still scanning the road.

When did you learn to do such tricks? It happened during infancy. You started to develop head control from the day you entered this world. Some time, around 4 months of age, you mastered it. You were able to move your head in all directions, and you were able to hold it still with your eyes level, regardless of the position of your body or the movements of your arms and legs.

How would your life be if you could not lift your head upwards and keep it there? You would not be able to look around and see where you were. You would only see the floor and your feet. The only place where you would be comfortable would be propped in a recliner, just the way an infant is propped in her infant seat.

Like Keith, children with milder forms of cerebral palsy start to hold their head in position without special treatment. Only later, when most infants typically crawl, sit, or stand, do these children with cerebral palsy require special intervention. Children with more serious developmental delay or cerebral palsy may not develop head control spontaneously and benefit from help as early as possible.

Meet Nina

Nina was born prematurely and diagnosed with cerebral palsy when she was three months old. Nina is small for her age and such a cutie. Her big smile and sparkling eyes charm everyone who meets her. Her mother, Pam, takes Nina in her infant seat for physical therapy. The treatment session proceeds nicely until the therapist starts to work on head control. These exercises are done in stomach-lying, a position Nina dislikes. Nina's smile fades away and she begins to cry. After three months and many therapy sessions, Nina still cries when placed on her stomach.

The therapist has given Nina's mother written home instructions and many suggestions on how to work with Nina, like propping her up on elbows while lying on her tummy (prone propping) on the floor, the diaper table, or a big ball. Nina doesn't like any of them. Everyone in the family, including Nina's grandparents, aunts, uncles, and friends are convinced that Nina simply will never want to be placed on her stomach. They reason that, just as some kids prefer vanilla while others prefer chocolate, Nina does not like to be on her stomach. It's just her preference. Since everyone, especially Pam, loves to see Nina happy, they have been avoiding the irritating stomach-lying position.

The therapist and Pam have failed to communicate effectively about Nina's dislike of being on her stomach. Pam follows all the therapy instructions that work on arm and hand movement and on rolling. She does them while Nina is side-lying or back-lying. Lying on her mother's lap or in her infant seat, Nina enjoys these activities. She is learning. Soon she can grasp and move a bright, colorful rattle. She can bring her hands together over her chest. With Pam's help, Nina begins to clap her hands. Soon she claps them all by herself. Nina loves to show off her new skills, and her family is delighted. In addition, Nina learns to roll, first from her side to her back, and then from her stomach to her back.

But the real question is, how much progress has Nina made with head control? After three more months of therapy, Nina can nod her head when she is in her infant seat. Yet, when placed on her tummy, she cannot lift her head and look around. Instead, she curls herself up, flips over onto her back, and happily plays in back-lying. When Nina is held upright or sits on her mom's lap, her head droops forward. She may bring it up briefly, but she is not able to keep it up for longer periods of time. After many months of weekly sessions, Nina has not acquired basic head control.

The once-friendly atmosphere of the treatment sessions becomes strained. The therapist is clearly frustrated. She has made little progress with her primary treatment goal for Nina to improve head control. She might blame herself. "My skills are not adequate. Despite my best efforts, I cannot help my patient achieve head control."

In therapy sessions, Nina tires quickly and cries easily. She cannot tolerate sustained physical activities that are challenging for her. Nina needs short exercise times interspersed throughout her day. Therapists know this and rely on parents to maintain a daily exercise home program.

The work done at home by the parents is most important, even more important than what the therapist does. Without follow-up at home, the exercises done during therapy time are like the proverbial "drop in the bucket." It evaporates before the next drop comes down. For children under two years of age, it is essential that at least one parent works with the child and carries out the recommended activities regularly. It is best when both parents work with the child. If neither of the parents is able or willing to do this, sadly, the weekly therapy sessions will be ineffective.

Pam has regularly worked with Nina and is generally happy with Nina's progress. Nina plays with toys, rolls over, and claps her hands. But Nina's head still droops forward when she is held up and Pam can't help but blame the therapist. "Why doesn't she just take care of it? After all, she is the professional. She should be able to get Nina to hold her head up."

Why has Nina shown so little progress with head control even after five months of therapy? Did the therapist use the wrong exercises or activities? Were the home instructions ill suited for Nina? Neither of these is true. The therapist selected just those activities that Nina needed. She gave good home instructions.

On the other hand, it is possible that Nina has such severe cerebral palsy, that, no matter what, she will never gain head control. Unfortunately, it is true that some children with cerebral palsy, regardless of how much the therapist and the parent work with them, will never master head control.

There were signs very early in her life that Nina had a significant defect within her nervous system. Fortunately, she was able to acquire some muscle control with persistent training. Therefore, we can reasonably assume that she also has the ability to slowly but surely acquire some basic head-holding skills, if given the right kind of exposure and training. ***The exercises proved ineffective because they were not used enough.*** The therapist worked with Nina once per week for an hour. This was simply not enough time for Nina to strengthen those muscles needed for adequate head control.

Does the entire fault rest on Nina's parents for not following the therapist's instruction for daily activities in the stomach-lying position? No; the truth is not so black and white. Nina cried in stomach-lying in therapy and at home. No one develops strong muscles and gains motor control by crying. Only when Nina is happy and motivated will she put forth the enormous effort needed to activate her muscles.

Motivation is the key! Motivation is everything! *Without motivation, children (all of us, for that matter) will not learn.* Therapists know this, and always tell parents to make home instruction fun for the child. Nina never had fun on her tummy, so she was never motivated to work in the position. Consequently, Pam no longer used the position at home.

Activities and exercises done in stomach-lying are the most effective approach to improving your child's head control. Disagreements on how much this position should be used are not helpful. *The therapist and the parent need to team up,* trying different ways to modify the activities until they find a way that is acceptable to the child. Only then can the training of head control get started. Pam may try inviting the extended family to participate in the effort. Attention and praise will go a long way to sustain Nina through her initial hard work. Abandoning the activity in therapy or at home is not an option if her parents want to help Nina.

Head-Up Practice

The *neck extensors* are the muscles that lift and hold our head up. They run along the back of the neck and are assisted by the upper portion of a large, flat back muscle called the trapezius (named for its trapezoid shape). The neck extensors work together with the back muscles.

Test this on yourself. Stretch out on your stomach with your head down. Put one hand on the back of your neck, and the other on your lower back. Lift your head and feel both your neck and your back muscles tightening. Next, lift your head only an inch off the surface and hold it there. You will feel the muscles getting taut. You are probably surprised how much work it requires to hold your head off the floor this small distance. Someone watching you might think you aren't doing anything at all. Now roll over onto your back, then again onto your stomach, and rest there. Notice that before you relaxed, you lifted your head and moved it into just the right spot for easy breathing and comfort.

What you just experienced provides you with a good strategy for strengthening your baby's neck muscles. Start each head control exercise with your baby stretched out on her tummy. Right after being placed in this position, your baby will most likely lift and move her head. Even lifting the head a small amount strengthens the muscles.

Initially, it is not at all important how high your baby lifts her head or how long the periods are that she spends on her tummy. You know that each time she tries to lift her head she is working. You shouldn't worry if she cries after spending a minute or even just 30 seconds on her tummy. Roll her out of the position and do it again later. Many short practice sessions will add up to a good work-out, and will strengthen your baby's neck muscles.

EASY HEAD-UP EXERCISES

These exercises will get your baby started. Let your physical therapist choose the ones that are best for your baby and you. Practice them with the therapist's help or supervision until you feel comfortable doing them at home.

Head-Up After Diaper Change

After a diaper change, roll your child onto her tummy with her head toward you. Bring her arms forward so her elbows are in front of her shoulders.

Lower yourself so you are at eye level with your child. Coax her with your voice, watch for slight head motions, and reward them. Make happy eye contact (photo 6.1).

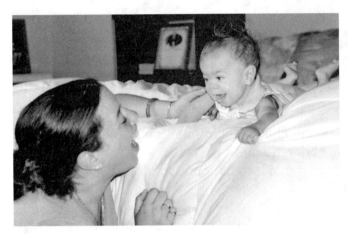

6.1

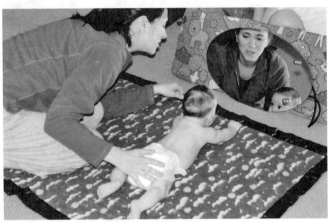

6.2

Head-Up on the Floor in Front of a Mirror

1. Place your baby on her tummy facing a mirror. Bring her arms forward so her elbows are in front of her shoulders.
2. Place your hand on her bottom and give some downward pressure. This will shift the weight from the upper body and make raising the head easier (photo 6.2). Observe her head, as well as her neck and back muscles. Any changes in these areas tell you if she is trying to lift her head.
3. Reward her with your voice or make happy eye contact using the mirror if her head comes up high enough.

Head-Up on You

1. Relax with your child in a comfortable back-lying position.
2. On her tummy prop your child up on your chest and secure her bottom (photo 6.3).
3. You are in a good position to notice any head-up movements and reward her efforts.

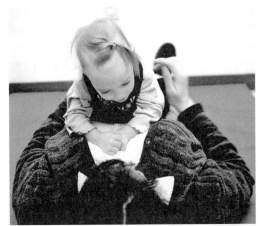

6.3

Head-Up on a Slanted Surface

When your child's head is higher than her body, the effect of gravity is reduced, making it easier to lift the head.

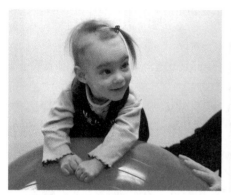

6.4

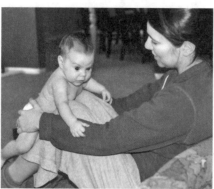

6.5

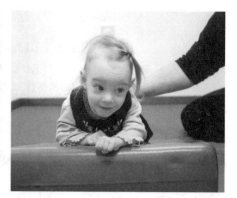

6.6

On an Exercise Ball

1. In front of a mirror, place your child on her tummy on a large exercise ball. Secure her by pressing her bottom against the ball.
2. Gently move the ball a little from side to side or forward and backwards. This will stimulate her to lift her head. (photo 6.4)
3. You are in a good position to notice all head-up efforts. Reward your child with words or happy eye contact using the mirror if her head comes up high enough.

On Your Legs

1. Sit relaxed against a comfortable back support. Bend your legs and place your baby on your lower legs facing you (photo 6.5).
2. Hold her well around her bottom.
3. Eye contact will be easy in this position. Reward her with a big smile as she brings her head up.

Note: Use this position only if your therapist recommends it. Do not use it if your child arches backwards or leans to one side.

On a Wedge

For this exercise, use a commercially available wedge, or use a couch cushion to make a slanted surface. Place the couch cushion on the floor and slant it by sliding two or three binders or telephone books of similar height in a row under one side of the cushion.

1. Place your child on her tummy on a wedge with her head at the highest end.
2. Sit in front of her, securing her shoulders and upper arms. Or if she props well on her forearms, be at her side and hold her bottom down (photo 6.6).
3. Talk and smile as she lifts her head.

Head-Up in Upright

Stand in front of a mirror. Hold your child facing away from you with one hand supporting her hips and the other hand supporting her chest (photo 6.7). Initially the child's chin may be supported as well. Encourage your child to lift her head up and look at herself in the mirror.

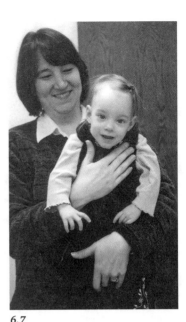

6.7

Head-Up with Wrinkles

When your child is working extra hard to bring her head up, horizontal wrinkles will appear on her forehead (photo 6.8). This is an indication that she is doing her best and deserves an extra big kiss afterwards.

After your child briefly lifts her head each time you place her on her tummy, you want her to hold her head up for longer periods of time. You want her to build up her endurance until one day she can hold it up for as long as she wants to.

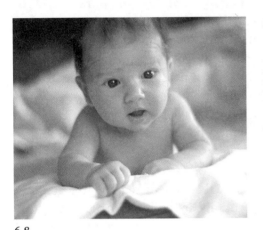

6.8

Head-Up Fun

Children work harder when they are having fun. Find out what your child enjoys most while being on her tummy. Will she hold her head up longer if you make funny sounds, sing, let a puppet talk to her (photo 6.9), or play peek-a-boo? For an older child, looking at her favorite book may encourage her to hold her head up longer.

Place your child on her tummy in a net swing. Hold her by her hands and gently swing her. Play "Where is my baby?" "Here she is!" you call out as she lifts her head and your eyes meet (photo 6.10).

Place your child on a scooter and secure her with a soft, wide strap. Holding onto her outstretched arms, pull her gently forward. An older child may hold onto a hoop and be pulled by it (photo 6.11).

Note: The last two activities are favorites of older children who still need to work on head control.

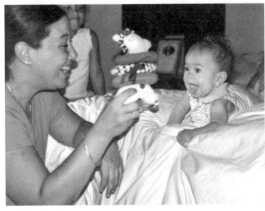

6.9

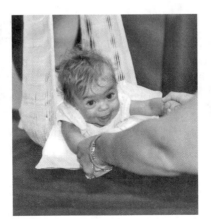

6.10

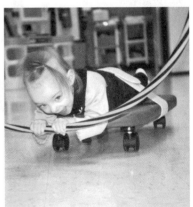

6.11

Integration of Head-Up Into Daily Life

All the extra effort and the exercises are wonderful to get your child started; to get her to understand and experience what she has to do to lift her head and hold it steady. By using the head-lifting and holding exercises described above, you are making a very difficult learning process easier by motivating and rewarding your child. Once your child has developed some head control by doing the exercises in this chapter, ***head-up needs to become part of an activity, part of each day, and part of life.*** For this to happen, your child needs to lift her head and hold it up, not for a reward but because she wants to. She needs to take over. She needs to make holding her head up part of her life. Asking her to lift her head and praising her if she does for months and months will hinder this process. Instead, as soon as possible, we want her to take ownership of her ability and incorporate it into her daily life.

This means drawing the child's attention to the task at hand. For instance, when Mom and Nina stretch out on the floor to look at a book together, Mom no longer coaxes her with: "Head up, Sugar!" Instead, she talks about the picture in the book. Once Nina raises her head, Mom accepts this is the normal thing to do and keeps on reading the story. If Nina holds her head up for 20 seconds, instead of 10 as before, Mom will be happy about it and smile, but will not talk about it. She is reading a book to Nina and wants her to stay focused on her story. ***This is what integration of head control into an activity means. No more requests to hold the head up, no more talk about it, and no more extra praising.***

The following are ways to integrate head-up into your child's routine.

- Every time after diapering, roll your child onto her stomach and let her stay in this position as long as it is convenient for you. You may have a little play routine you like to do with her, or she can lie there while you straighten up the diaper table.

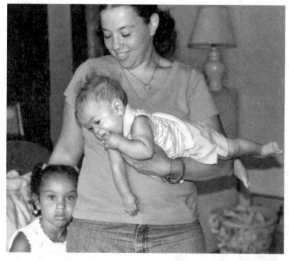

6.12

- Every time you place her on the floor, put her on her stomach first. Never mind that she will soon flip over on her back, or fusses and you will then turn her over on her back. Regardless, always put her on her stomach first.
- Every time you pick her up from back-lying, put her on her stomach first, let her stay there a short time and then pick her up.
- Every time you carry your child, have her face away from you with her trunk leaning slightly forward, as is shown in photo 6.7.
- Try carrying your child in stomach-lying (photo 6.12). Observe whether your child intermittently lifts and holds her head, or at least tries to lift her head. If so, use this mode of carrying her when it is convenient for you.

Your Child Practices Head-Up Independently

Find some toys that are interesting for your child to watch and listen to. Use them only for this activity.

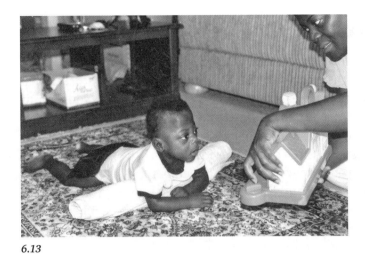
6.13

Place your child on her stomach with a rolled-up towel under her chest. The towel roll will lift her chest off the floor and ensure that she is propped up on her elbows and that they are under or in front of the shoulders. Drape a five-pound ankle weight over your child's buttocks. (A sock filled with rice or dry beans and tied shut also makes a good weight.) This will help to straighten the hips and shift the body weight backwards, making it easier to lift the head.

Hold a toy up for her to watch (photo 6.13).

Next, choose a music box (or similar toy that moves and makes sounds), place it in front of your child, and walk away. Or you may put on a video or DVD to encourage her to look up. Even if she lifts her head only briefly once or twice to look and listen, it's a start of independent play in stomach-lying. *It's the start of independent, integrated head control.* Stop the activity as soon as your child fusses.

Note: Do not encourage your child to use her hands during this activity. Don't tell her to touch the toy. Stretching and reaching with the arms makes lifting the head more difficult. Instead, encourage your child to remain propped on her elbows and enjoy watching and listening. Without moving, it will be easier for her to hold her head up.

Head-Up on a Boppy Pillow

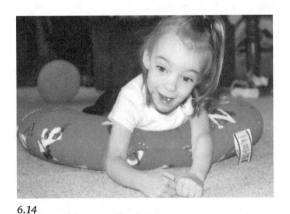
6.14

Placed on a Boppy pillow, a bigger child may enjoy being on her tummy and holding her head up while propping on elbows (photo 6.14). It's a good position to hang out, watch what's going on, and exercise the neck, upper back, and shoulder muscles at the same time. (A Boppy pillow is a curved firm pillow, which is available in stores with baby items, many general stores, and even some drugstores.)

Use of a Prone Stander

For an older child who still needs to work on head control, use a prone stander as much as possible. With the stander set in a forward leaning position, the child will exercise her neck and upper back muscles. With the stander set in an upright position, basic head holding skills will be reinforced. In preschool, your child can be in a prone stander during story time and during one-on-one instructions (photo 6.15). At home, she can be in the prone stander when looking at books, watching TV, etc. (photo 6.16).

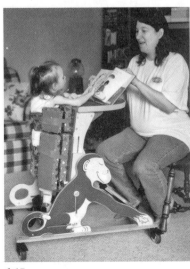
6.15

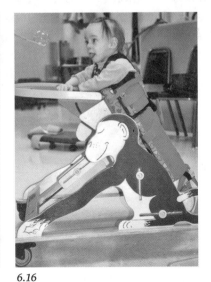
6.16

Frequently Asked Questions by Parents

Q. *"How often should I do the head-up exercises with my child?"*
A. All the time. Well, no. Your therapist most likely will give you sensible directions. "Please try to do this three to four times a day." Considering how much your infant sleeps during the day and how much time feedings take, this is a good schedule. You want to catch those times when your child feels well, is not hungry, and is rested, active, and alert. There are usually three or four periods during the day that fit that description, and this is when you want to practice. Remember, initially it is not important how high or how long your child lifts her head. If she fusses, roll her over, give her a minute of rest, and then try again. All those short practices will add up to a good exercise session.

Q. *"When will I see improvement and what are some of the signs of progress?"*
A. All the time. Of course, there will be variations. Sometimes your child will not do as well as at other times. But overall, there will be a steady trend of progress. It will start to take less time, less coaxing, and less extra effort on your part for your child to lift her head. The head will come up higher. It will come up straighter—with her eyes level. She will be able to hold her head up longer. First she may hold it up only seconds longer. Yet, each second counts. Observe what she does when her head is up. Does she look around? Does she look at you? Does she smile? All these are signs of progress. This first intensive work on a new skill is exciting and rewarding.

Q. *"How long should I do the head-up exercises? Days? Weeks? Months?"*
A. As short a time as possible. "Why only for a short time if it is helping?" Your goal is for your child to hold her head up all the time, not just when she exercises. To achieve this I recommend that you fade out the exercises as soon as possible and follow the recommendations of *Integration of Head-up into Daily Life*.

Q. *"Why is integration of head control so important?"*
A. Head control is an automatic response. We do it without thinking about it. When we move, our head position changes without us paying any attention to it. Yes, if we want to, we can pay attention to the positions or movements of our head. But usually we don't even think about it. You hold your head up all day long. Can you remember when you did it consciously? I bet you can't, and this is my point. As soon as possible, you want your child to hold her head as automatically as you do.

7

Happy Baby in Back-lying

There is a yoga pose called "happy baby." It is easy to do. You lie on your back, stick your arms and legs up in the air, and enjoy. That's it—happy baby. It mimics how babies spend their first happy hours in play. They look at their hands and watch as they move. Their hands touch; they feel it and are fascinated by the sensation. Their legs come up, they touch their feet, and their world is full of wonder.

In this position, the muscles that are working are in the front of the body. They bend the joints and are called flexor muscles. It is in this back-lying position that infants learn their first functional skill—putting hands to mouth. Even if parents don't want them to, babies succeed in sucking their fingers or their thumb. You may regard it as a nuisance. But think about it. Isn't this the first step toward self-feeding? Eating independently is a very important skill.

Full-term infants can do this hand-to-mouth movement very early because they are born with their arm and leg joints slightly bent. This is called *physiological flexion of the newborn.* It gives them an advantage that makes bending the arm easy. Babies are born this way because they have spent the last months before delivery curled up in the cramped space of their mother's womb. It is easier to bend your shoulder or hip joint if you start out from an already mildly bent position.

Try to experience this yourself. Lie stretched out on your back so that all parts of your arms and legs touch the floor and then lift your arms and legs up into the air. Try it again, but bend your legs and arms a bit before you raise them. You will notice that it is easier with your limbs slightly bent.

Infants who are born at 29 weeks or earlier show little or no physiological flexion at birth. By the time their nervous system has matured enough to allow voluntary movements in back-lying, they have a harder time doing them than full-term babies.

There is another hurdle for premies to overcome. In back-lying, their immature nervous system causes an increase of the muscle tone of their back muscles (extensor tone). Their back is straight and stiff, their shoulders are pulled back, and their legs are stretched out. This makes bending the shoulders and hips even more difficult. Consequently, premies may not start playing with hands and feet as early as they should.

Infants born with very low muscle tone and infants born with increased extensor tone due to a defect of the nervous system show a similar delay of hand-to-mouth, hand-to-hand, or hand-to-foot play.

Happy Baby Exercises

For children who need help acquiring early play skills in back-lying, physical therapists may recommend some or all of the following activities. The first three are *passive range of motion* exercises. They are called passive because the children do not move on their own but the parent curls up the child's trunk or lifts and moves his arms for him. The exercises are meant to loosen your child's joints and muscles, mildly stretch them, and allow him to experience normal movement patterns.

Technique is important when you do passive movements with your child. For instance, when you do *Moving One Arm at a Time,* your child's shoulder joints needs to be in a good position—not pulled up or back. Therefore, the shoulder joint is placed just right, stabilized with one hand, and only then the arm is moved. Keeping your child's muscle tone and his body size in mind, the therapist will show you where and how to place your hand to stabilize the shoulder joint. Be sure to practice the exercises first with the therapist before you do them at home. The written instructions will then be a reminder for you. They are not sufficient on their own.

The first exercise is meant to loosen and mildly stretch your child's back muscles and the muscles around the shoulder blades.

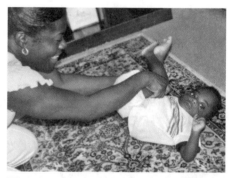

7.1

Spine Curl-Up

Your child lies on his back. Grasp under his upper legs and curl him into a "ball" so his bottom is up in the air. Roll him slowly to the right, then to the left and then back down (photo 7.1).

Moving One Arm at a Time

This activity will help you loosen your child's shoulder muscles and stimulate arm movements.

1. Your child lies on his back. Slide your right hand under his left shoulder so your fingers rest on top of the shoulder and your thumb wraps around it (photo 7.2).

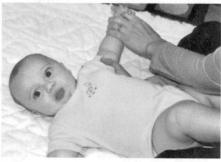

7.2

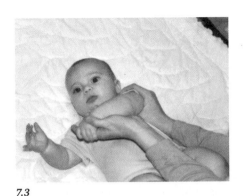

7.3

2. Gently pull the shoulder down in the direction of the feet. Bend the arm at the shoulder.
3. Holding his left hand with your left hand, move his arm toward the opposite shoulder as far as it goes without pulling the arm (photo 7.3), and then move it back out to the side.
4. Repeat five times with each arm.

If your child's shoulder joints do not need to be stabilized, the therapist may recommend that you move both arms at the same time as shown and explained below. This is done at three different speeds. At the slow speed, you move the arms through their full range of motion and mildly stretch the arm muscles. At the faster speeds, you move the arms as far as they go with ease, which will not be less than their full range. The faster movements do not stretch the arm muscles. They are just meant to loosen them. Do **not** do the faster movements if your child tenses his arm when you do them.

When you do the three arm movements, make sure you look at and talk to your child. *Happy eye contact encourages your child to keep his head in the middle* and not flop it from side to side.

Three Arm Movements

Your child lies on his back facing you. Hold his hands by placing your thumbs into his palms. Let the tips of your thumbs rest between his thumbs and index fingers and loosely wrap your other fingers around his hands and wrists.

Boxing

1. Gently pull the right arm up until the elbow is straight. Pause (figure 7.4).
2. Gently push the arm down while you pull the left arm up until the elbow is straight. Pause.
3. Repeat two times.
4. Next, repeat the boxing motion at a faster speed, and then do it very fast.

Out and Over

1. Gently pull both arms up until the elbows are straight.
2. Slowly swing the arms out to the sides. Pause (figure 7.5a).
3. Slowly swing the arms up and cross them over the chest. Pause (figure 7.5b).
4. Repeat two times.
5. Next, do it at a faster speed, and then at a very fast speed.

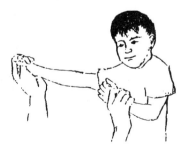

7.4

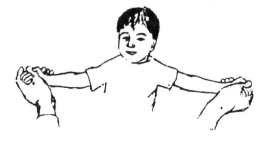

7.5a

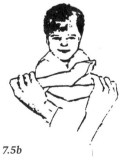

7.5b

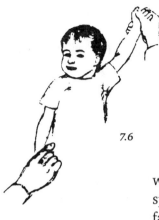

Windmill

1. Gently pull both arms up until the elbows are straight.
2. Slowly swing one straight arm up beside the head and the other arm down beside the trunk. Pause (figure 7.6).
3. Now move the arms until their positions are reversed. Pause.
4. Repeat two times.
5. Next, do it at a faster speed, and then at a fast speed.

7.6

To do all three movements after each diaper change does not take long. It is time well spent. Most babies like them very much, especially if you change the movement speed as recommended. They like it if you move slow - pause - slow - pause -, faster, faster, faster, faster, and then fast/fast/fast/fast/. If your child did not smile before, by fast/fast/fast/fast he will surely giggle! Talking or singing while you do the movements makes them even more fun.

If your child enjoys the three arm movements, you may notice that he does not remain passive but participates with the movements, which will be very good.

Note: Remember—do the arm movements only at a slow speed if your child does not like the fast movements and tenses his arms.

Happy Baby Plays with You

Now your child is ready to play.

Your child lies on your lap facing you. Cradle both shoulders with your hands. Smile at him and bring his hands to your face by bending his arms at the shoulder and

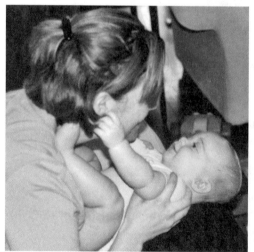

holding them up (photo 7.7). Have him touch your cheeks, mouth, and so on. You may tell him what he is touching—"that's mama's ear." Your child's head should be in the middle (the eyes are level) as he looks and listens to your baby talk. You may play patty-cake or peek-a-boo with him or what ever comes to mind.

Next, bring his legs up as you did for the spine curl-up, and have his feet touch your face. Play with him as long as he enjoys it.

Variation: When your child is familiar with the play situation, encourage him to do more on his own. Help him bend his arms at the shoulders, talk to him, and see if he touches you. If he does not, move his arms up and place his hands on your cheeks or mouth. See if he will keep them there for a few seconds when you no longer support his arms.

7.7

Happy Baby Plays with Feet

Once your baby can bring his arms up and his hands together, he is ready for this activity.

1. Your baby lies on your lap facing you. Talk to him as you grasp under his upper legs, and bring them up.
2. Encourage him to touch his knees or feet. If he cannot do this, hold his right leg up with your left hand, and, with your right hand, support his left upper arm as much as necessary for him to be able to touch his legs (photo 7.8).
3. Repeat this and help your child touch his left leg with his right hand. Play as long as your baby enjoys it.

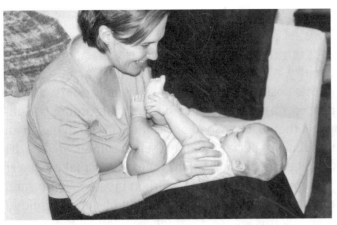

7.8

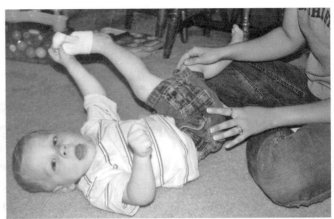

7.9

Variation:

1. Your child lies on the floor. By pushing up his seat you make it easy for him to lift one leg with knees turned out.
2. Encourage him to touch his foot and pull off his sock with the opposite hand or both hands (photo 7.9). If needed, help him to grab onto the sock and then let him pull it off on his own.
3. Repeat with the opposite leg and arm.

Colorful socks or booties with bells on them provide variety and an extra incentive to bring up the hands and feet for play.

Independent Play In Back-Lying

Now your baby may be ready to play by himself. Follow your physical therapist's directions on how to position him on his back.

When your child plays in back-lying, you want his head centered between his shoulders, his trunk straight, his arms bent at the shoulders, and his legs bent at the hips.

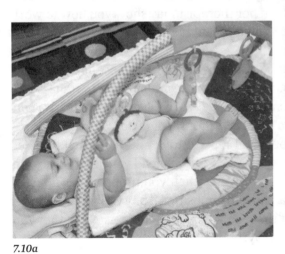

7.10a

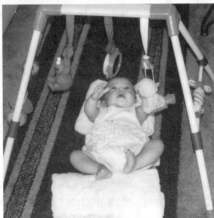

7.10b

Roll up a towel from each side, turn it over, and place your baby between the towel rolls. In photo 7.10a, the towel rolls are alongside the baby's body for support and to help bend the arms at the shoulders. The baby's head is placed on a folded diaper so it is in the middle with the chin tucked. In photo 7.10b, the towel rolls are alongside the head and shoulders to discourage the child from turning her head and to slightly bend the arms at the shoulders. A bigger towel roll is placed under the legs against the baby's bottom. This helps the baby bend her legs at the hip.

Place a baby gym over your child. The dangling toys will entice him to reach up with his arms and to lift his feet.

Is Your Child Ready for Back-lying

Lying on their back by themselves during their waking hours is not a good position for many children with cerebral palsy. Abnormal reflexes and abnormal muscle tone will affect the children more in this position. In back-lying they may not be able to bring their hands together for play or roll over onto their sides or their tummies. Consequently, they will not be happy on their backs. Good positioning in side-lying, in an infant seat, car seat, reclining high chair, a specially adapted seat recommended by the therapist, or in a prone stander will be more beneficial for them. It will make it easier for them to play and socialize with people. It also protects their muscles, joints, and bones. If your child's physical therapist recommends that you not place your child in the back-lying position for play, follow this advice. Chapter 3 explained the reasons for these precautions against back-lying.

Note: The happy baby activities may also be done with your child lying in an infant or car seat. If needed, support your child's head and body with a folded diaper and a rolled-up towel as described above. You want your child's head in the middle, his shoulders level, and his trunk straight. If your child slouches to one side in the seat, avoid using it as much as possible unless your child's therapist can help you solve the problem.

Frequently Asked Questions By Parents

Q. *"Emily is 6 months old. She likes to play in back-lying, but when I pull her to sitting, her head flops back if I don't support it. I am very worried about this, but Emily's therapist doesn't seem concerned. She is pleased that Emily holds her head up when I carry her and when she sits on my lap. She says Emily is making good progress. What do you think?"*
A. Emily has mastered two very important skills. She holds her head in upright and she plays in back-lying. Next, you want Emily to be able to lift and hold her head when she is on her tummy. After she masters this, her therapist may show you how to work with Emily so she learns to hold her head when pulled up from back-lying.

Q. *"Abby likes to play in back-lying. When she was smaller, I propped her up with towels and she touched the dangling toys of the baby gym with either hand. Now that she is bigger and propping her up with towels no longer works, I observe her using only her right hand and she frequently turns her head to the side. What should I do?"*
A. What you describe indicates that abnormal muscle tone and abnormal reflexes are interfering with Abby's arm movements. When Abby's head was in midline and her shoulders were slightly rounded—as they were when you propped her up with towels—this happened less. Since you can no longer position Abby well in back-lying, use the position only for short periods of time. Talk to Abby's therapist. Together you will find better ways to position Abby for playtime.

Q. *"My son Chris is a year old. In back-lying, he has started to scoot around on the floor. His therapist does not want him to do this. Why? Isn't it good that he is learning to move around on his own?"*
A. Yes, it is good that he moves around. But his therapist is right, nevertheless. It is not good for Chris to scoot around on his back. It does not teach him coordination

and does not strengthen his muscles for other skills that he will need to learn. I am sure you want Chris to learn to roll over, crawl, sit up, stand, and walk. Scooting on his back does not help him to acquire any of these abilities.

Once scooting on his back becomes a habit for Chris, it may even hinder him from learning other ways of moving about. When scooting on his back, Chris pushes his shoulders backward. When rolling over, however, the shoulders need to be pulled forward—just the opposite of what he is doing. When he sits or stands, pushing the shoulders back can cause him to fall backwards and prevent him from regaining his balance.

Please, follow your therapist's advice. The sooner Chris learns to move about by rolling or crawling, the better it will be for his motor development. Placing Chris on his tummy will keep him from scooting. It will encourage him to use his muscles in ways that will help his motor skill development. If Chris does not like to be on his tummy, follow suggestions and activities given in Chapters 6 and 8, which may help him to like the position.

8

Tummy Time

Starting in the early 1990s, pediatricians in the United States began recommending that infants sleep on their back. This directive has gradually reduced the incidence of SIDS (Sudden Infant Death Syndrome). It also has reduced the time infants spent on their stomach. As a remedy, physicians ask parents to give their infants "tummy time" during the day when they are awake.

This is good advice. As explained in Chapter 3, the amount of time your baby spends on her stomach makes a difference. In stomach-lying, infants start to use the muscles of the backside of their body, the extensor muscles. These are the muscles that typically are weak in children with developmental delay or with cerebral palsy. Therefore, *tummy time is especially important for children with gross motor delays or with cerebral palsy.*

A good way to start tummy time is outlined in Chapter 6, Head-Up. Place your child on her tummy throughout the day for brief periods again and again so that she gets used to the position.

The first battle will be won when your child, after being placed on her tummy, contentedly looks around. She may, however, not like to be on her tummy for long periods because just looking around gets boring pretty quickly. Before your child will be happy in this position for any length of time, she needs to be able to play on her tummy, interact with toys, and have fun.

"Playing in tummy-lying is easy. Babies love it." This is what everyone believes. But is it true? Find out for yourself. Stretch out on the floor and pretend to play like a baby. After a few minutes, you will know that it is hard work. A great deal of upper body strength and arm coordination is required. Children with cerebral palsy or similar movement disorders need much practice to master it.

Prerequisites for Tummy Time with Play

What are the necessary components that make it possible for a child to play on her tummy, or in prone position, as your therapist may call it?

Easy Head-Up. The higher your child can lift her head, the easier it is for her to hold it up. Plain physics is involved. If the head is lifted 45 degrees, its center of mass (weight as acted on by gravity) is in front of the shoulders and muscle strength is required to keep it up. Once the head is lifted 90 degrees, the weight of the head rests over the shoulders and little effort is needed to keep it there.

A child who is able to bring her head all the way up may do so to rest and relax her neck muscles during play. A child who can lift it up only 45 degrees has to put her head down when she gets tired. As long as your child still needs to intermittently put her head down and rest, it is only safe for her to play with soft toys while on her tummy.

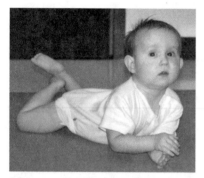
8.1

Propping Up on Elbows and Forearms. Did you ever see an old-fashioned baby picture with the baby propped up on a fur rug? This is exactly what you want your baby to do. When your child is solidly propped up on both elbows, she is ready to take her hands off the surface and touch something. While her elbows stay propped, she will be able to cradle the toy between her hands (see photo 8.1).

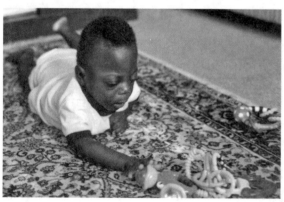
8.2

Propping Up on One Forearm. For more interesting play, babies do not just touch the rattle. They turn it, shake it, drop it, and reach for it. To do so, they take one arm off the surface. For successful play with one arm, the weight of the upper body is first shifted over one forearm, which frees the other arm to reach and play (photo 8.2). ***This weight shift and propping up on one forearm is a challenging task for many children with cerebral palsy.*** Some acquire the skill slowly on their own by spending lots of time on their tummies. Others need extra help to learn the task, and for some it may always be difficult.

Exercises for Tummy Time with Play

The first two tummy exercises help to prepare your child to shift her weight, reach, and play in stomach-lying. They do not take long and are easy to do if your child is used to spending some time in stomach-lying. Practicing them with a child who does not like to be on her stomach is a different story. If your child is not used to being on her stomach, start the exercises very gradually. Begin with just the first exercise, *Rocking on Forearms*. Do the activity only as long as your child likes it. If she fusses after 10 seconds, do it only 10 seconds. To make up for the short time, do it as often as you can manage or what works for you: Each time before and after you change her diaper, each time before you pick her up, before and after her nap and so on. If you work outside the home, you may even ask your baby sitter or daycare worker to do it.

Keep doing the routine until your child likes it when you rock her on forearms. Now you may expand her tummy time. After *Rocking on Forearms* do *Rocking and Reach* with her. If she is happy and alert after both exercises you may follow the recommendations of *Independent Tummy Time Cradling Toys* and have her spend some more time on her tummy.

Use the exercises as directed by your child's physical therapist and follow any specific directions given.

Rocking on Forearms

1. On the changing table, on your bed, or on the floor, help your child to roll onto her tummy facing you.
2. Support her upper arms so her elbows are under or slightly in front of her shoulders.
3. Gently rock your child from one forearm to the other. Do it as you sing or play a little song for rhythm and fun (photo 8.3).

Do this several times a day.

After your child is used to the exercise, reduce your support to her upper arms. Instead, with your open hands lightly touch the arm and shoulder as you rock her side to side.

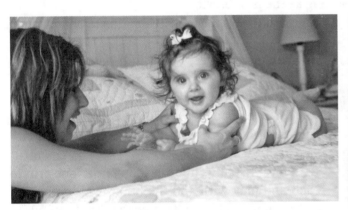

8.3

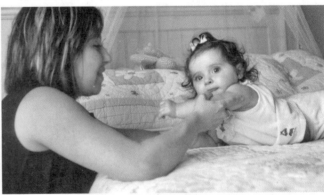

8.4

Rocking and Reach

1. Start with rocking on forearms, as described above.
2. Next, lean your child all the way over to the right forearm—rock—and, supporting the upper arm and elbow, stretch the left arm out—reach (photo 8.4).
3. Place the left forearm back on the surface. Then lean her all the way over to the left forearm—rock—and stretch out the right arm—reach.

Do ten repetitions several times a day.

Try to create a rhythm. A steady rhythm and saying "rock - and - reach" will help your child to know what to expect and to participate.

Independent Tummy Time Cradling Toys

Is your child ready for some independent play on her tummy? Positioning her as explained here will make it easier. First do this with the help of your therapist and follow any specific directions given.

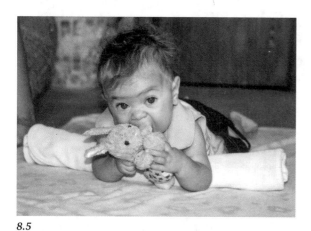

8.5

1. Place your child on her stomach with a roll (rolled-up receiving blanket or towel) under her chest so her elbows are positioned under or slightly in front of her shoulders.
2. Place a five-pound ankle weight or sandbag over her buttocks. (This will help straighten the hips and shift the bodyweight backwards, making it easier for her to hold her head up.)
3. Set a soft toy between her hands for independent play (photo 8.5). See the Appendix for tips on making your own sandbags.

Have your child play like this several times a day.

Tummy Time with Reach

1. Position your child as described in the above activity.
2. Stretch out in front of her with an interesting toy. Support her left elbow, help her to lean over to the left, and wait for her to reach for the toy with her right hand.
3. If your child does not reach out for the toy, place her hand on it and let her figure out what to do.
4. Later, support the right elbow while your child reaches with her left hand.
5. Have your child play as long as she is interested.

If your child has hemiplegia have her always reach with her affected hand when you practice with her.

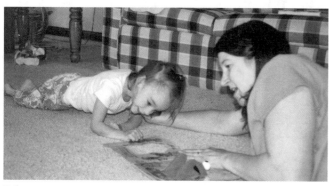

8.6

Variation: After your child has shown some progress, try the activity without propping her up with a towel roll or using the weights (photo 8.6).

For an older child who still benefits from *Tummy Time with Reach,* use an age appropriate activity instead of a toy.

Note: Usually children soon prefer one arm to reach and play with and the other arm to prop up on. For many reasons, it is important that your child learn to prop or play with either arm. Continue the assisted play in stomach-lying until your child can play independently with either hand.

What's Next?

After your child is able to play in stomach-lying, she will like the position. When placed on her back, she will roll over, and if she cannot do so, she won't be happy until you help her to get onto her tummy. As your child spends more and more time on her tummy, her arms, shoulders, and upper body muscles will become more coordinated. She will learn to stretch her arm far forward, reach to the side, turn to the side, and maybe even scoot backward or forward. Progress is now relatively easy and fast.

Yet, even with plenty of time on her tummy, a child with cerebral palsy may not learn all the skills she needs unless she receives special help. Sean's story, below, shows how this help may be soundly rejected by the child.

Big Push-Ups for Sean

Sean is eighteen months old. He is a clever, busy little guy. Sean has a diagnosis of cerebral palsy and has been receiving physical therapy for a year. Today his mom brings him to his session. She puts Sean down and proudly tells the therapist that Sean is learning his colors. The therapist is impressed. As the adults talk, Sean seizes the moment. He quickly rolls on his tummy. Ready to play, he scans the room. "Hmm—what's interesting around here?" Oh yes, he likes the Sesame Street pop-up toy. Off he goes, pulling himself forward with both arms, digging his little elbows into the carpet. The left knee also comes forward and helps with the forward lunge. It is not easy to drag crawl (also called commando crawling). You can try it and find out. You may run out of breath pretty quickly. Sean sure knows how to make a go of it. He pauses, looks at Mom, and his expression says: "Aren't I doing great?" "Yes, you are, Sweetie," Mom's proud smile answers.

Sean just learned to drag crawl. Three months ago he had been barely able to move a bit to the side. Moving forward is so good; it's liberating. Sean is no longer helplessly immobile. He moves and explores. He is eagerly using his new skills. The therapist is pleased with Sean's progress. Independent mobility is so very important for a child's overall development. Not surprisingly, Sean is making progress in other areas too. But, of course, there are better ways to move about than drag crawling. It is the therapist's job to improve and build up the gross motor skills of his or her little patients. This is the purpose of the therapy session.

The therapist moves Sean's right leg up after he has pushed off with his left as he takes off again. She is helping him learn to crawl reciprocally. At least this is her intention. When reciprocally commando crawling, children push off with one elbow and the opposite knee. It teaches them to move the right leg together with the left arm and the left leg with the right arm. Doing so, children learn an alternating, coordinated movement pattern with their arms and legs. This is something new that will prepare them for crawling on hands and knees and for walking.

When reciprocally commando crawling, the body lifts slightly off the floor, and moving forward becomes easier than when the tummy brushes the floor. Sean thinks differently. "This does not help me at all!" He stops in his tracks. No more crawling for now. No coaxing by Mom or the therapist helps. Sean has made up his mind. "Either I do it my way or no way!" The therapist does not get the message. Next she puts him on hands and knees. "Oh no, not this again!" Now Sean is really upset. He cries, his arms give, his legs stretch out. He has had it!

Why doesn't Sean like to be on his hands and knees? Does the position hurt him? No, most likely he cries because he feels unsafe in this position. Most likely he feels afraid that he could fall on his face at any moment. His arms are too weak to hold him up. Even with the therapist's assistance, he is not sure he can stay up. Also, keeping his legs bent is hard for him. When he lifts his head, all his extensor muscles are working. Unfortunately, the extensor muscles of his legs want to work too. They straighten his legs and make him drop down onto his tummy.

For Sean, being on hands and knees probably feels as risky and unsafe as you would if someone asked you to stand and balance on a moving ball. "Why would I do that?" you ask.

All stretched out on the floor and propped up on his elbows, Sean feels comfortable. He can lift his head, he can play, he can move—it is fun. Why would he want to do something different?

A typically developing seven- or eight-month-old infant who has just started to move forward on his tummy does not mind being placed on his hands and knees. Months earlier when he played on his tummy, he had pushed up to "big arms," gaining strength and control of the muscles that hold the elbow straight. Sean skipped this developmental "exercise." He progressed from elbow propping to moving to the side on elbows, and now to crawling with elbow push-off. But he has never straightened both elbows and pushed to a big-arm position.

Sean has a type of cerebral palsy that increases the tone of the muscles that bend the elbows, thereby making it hard for him to straighten the elbows. When he was younger and played in back-lying, he kept his arms close to his chest. It took special effort and much prompting to get him to reach up high, and usually he never fully stretched out his elbows. Playing on his tummy, he was eager to reach far, and with time became able to fully stretch out his left arm. But he can only partially straighten out his right elbow. Children like Sean need much extra work and training to gain strength and control of their shoulder and arm muscles, especially of their triceps muscles.

The triceps is the muscle that runs along the back of your upper arm from your shoulder to your elbow. You can feel your left triceps when you run your right hand over the back of your straightened upper left arm. Squeeze it and feel how big it is. Rest the weight of your upper body on your arm or lean on your straight arm and feel how your triceps works hard to keep your arm stable.

For Sean to progress in crawling, his triceps muscles need to become stronger and more coordinated. Bearing weight on straight arms is a key component of many skills. Once Sean can push himself into a big-arm position, many new possibilities will open up to him. He may push to a hands-and-knees position, start crawling on hands and knees, and push into sitting. Bearing weight on big arms will also help him learn to stretch out his arms as he protects himself when falling.

In summary, strengthening Sean's triceps muscles is a top priority at his physical therapy sessions as well as his home program.

"Big Arm" Exercises

If your child is at risk for cerebral palsy and shows tightness of her arm muscles, it makes sense not to wait, but to stimulate elbow straightening—work of the triceps muscles—early on. Chapter 7 describes the range of motion exercises: *Three Arm movements*. Doing these exercises after each diaper change encourages your child to straighten her arms with your help in an easy and fun way. The movements mildly stretch the biceps muscles as well as stimulate the triceps muscle to work.

Shoulder – Elbow – Hand

This exercise is a good way to strengthen the triceps muscle early on without getting the baby upset. If your therapist suggests that you do the exercise with your child, carefully observe her demonstrating it. Your child may want to pull her shoulders backwards during the exercise and the therapist will show you how to prevent this from happening.

1. Your child lies on her back facing you.

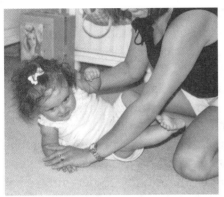

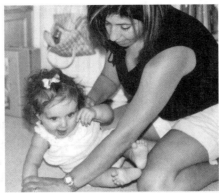

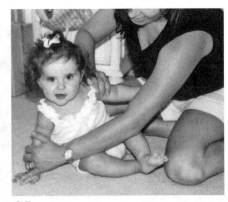

8.7a   8.7b   8.7c

2. Hold your child by the left upper arm, roll her to the right and lift her so that she comes to rest first on her right shoulder, then up onto her right elbow, finally pressing down on her hand (photo 8.7a, 8.7b).
3. The elbow is now straight and the weight of her upper body rests on it. With your free hand, support the elbow as needed.
4. Have your child prop herself up like this for 5 to 10 seconds (photo 8.7c).
5. Ease her into back-lying the same way she came up. Change hands and do the same with the other arm.

Do this exercise several times a day. If your child has hemiplegia, always practice with her affected arm.

Variation. As your child gets used to the exercise you may start to pull her up by the hand instead of holding onto her shoulder. It is a sign of progress if she stays on the straight arm with less support to the elbow.

Note: The Shoulder-Elbow-Hand exercise is not a preparation for sitting up. Small children do not sit up from back-lying. They roll over onto their stomach and then push into sitting.

Independent Play in Back-Lying

Have your child play in back-lying as recommended in Chapter 7. After she shows interest in playing with the toys, start hanging them a little higher. This will encourage her to straighten her elbows as she plays.

Weight Bearing on "Big Arms"

Fully straightening both arms is a good skill, but being able to keep them straight while bearing weight on them is even more useful. Therapists practice weight bearing on both arms in a variety of ways. They work on the floor, over a roll, on a ball, over a wedge, and may even use suspended equipment. They choose the equipment to make weight bearing on straight arms easier, more interesting, more challenging, or just more fun for the child. According to your child's needs and what works best, the physical therapist will give you specific instructions for you to use at home.

The next exercises are examples for weight bearing on straight arms. They do not take long. Do them several times each day as directed by your child's therapist and follow any specific instructions given.

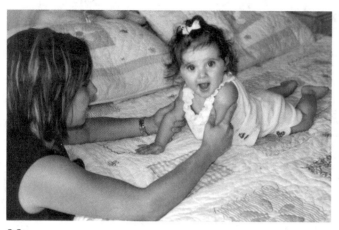

8.8a

Rocking on Big Arms

1. Have your child lie on her stomach, preferably on a higher surface such as the diaper table or a firm bed, facing you.
2. Grasp around your child's upper arms and elbows, and help her to come up, straighten her elbows, and bear weight on her hands.
3. Loosen your grasp. Preferably, you support just the back of the elbows as little as needed while you gently rock your child from side to side. Talk to her or sing while you do this (photo 8.8a).

Do this several times a day.

The rocking motion causes a slight weight shift from one arm to the other. This makes the exercise easier, more effective, and closer to real-life situations.

Variation: If your child is older and bigger, put a folded-up beach towel, a firm pillow, or a Boppy pillow under her chest (figure 8.8b). With the chest lifted up, less weight is on the arms and straightening them is easier.

Note: If your child's arms muscles are weak or spastic, your therapist may recommend that your child wear soft elbow splints initially during this and the following two exercises.

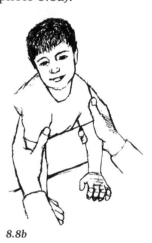

8.8b

Big Arm Taps

The next two exercises are similar to the one before and are done in the same position. When your therapist decides that your child is ready for them, you may add them to the "Rocking on Big Arms" practice.

The first exercise requires your child to make a brief, complete weight shift from one arm to the other. It helps her practice the arm movements necessary for crawling. Later, when your child is ready for crawling, this training will pay off.

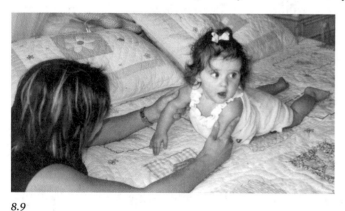

8.9

1. Place your child on her stomach.
2. Grasp around your child's upper arms and elbows and help her come up, straighten her elbows, and bear weight on her hands.
3. Talk to your child, encouraging her to lift her head and feel secure and confident.
4. Next, help her lean toward her right arm. Now lift her left hand about an inch off the surface, and then let it drop down—tap (photo 8.9). Help her lean toward her left arm, lift her right hand about an inch off the surface, and let it drop down—tap.

Repeat 10 times several times a day.

Big Arm Touchdown

This exercise encourages a quick response from the shoulder and arm muscles, especially the triceps muscles. It will build strength in the triceps and will trigger

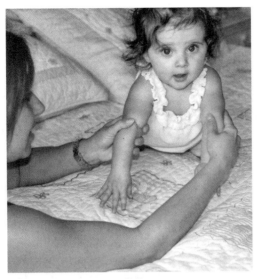 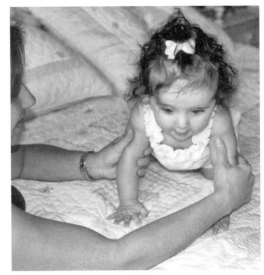

8.10a *8.10b*

immediate muscle activation. A quick response from the triceps muscles keeps the elbow straight when you fall forward. The Big Arm touchdowns are early training for catching oneself from a fall with outstretched arms.

1. Practice as before but instead of lifting just one hand, lift both hands about 2 inches off the surface, and then let them both touch down. Pause (photos 8.10a, 8.10b).
2. Repeat.

Do 10 repetitions several times a day.

Variation: When your child is used to the exercise, try to lift her arms a little higher and then let them tap down. If the hands fist or turn over with the touchdown, lift them less.

Note: *The exercises will help your child only if done daily for several weeks.* Just doing them occasionally will not make a difference. You may follow the *Shoulder-Arm Workout* routine to make the exercises fun for you and your child.

Shoulder-Arm Workout

This is for a child who cannot yet hold herself up on hands and knees. Ask your therapist if your child is ready for this workout. It combines the previous exercises in a pleasant sequence.

1. Put on some music you and your child enjoy.
2. Place your child on her tummy on a comfortable firm surface such as your bed.
3. Sit or kneel in front of your child and do exercises:
   - Rocking on Forearms
   - Rocking and Reach
   - Rocking on Big Arms
   - Big Arm Taps
   - Big Arm Touchdowns
   - Shoulder-Elbow-Hand

Start out doing the exercises at a slow pace for only 4 to 6 repetitions each. Make it fun. Stop if your child fusses or complains. When your child is used to the routine, do more repetitions of the exercises. Do the workout session two times daily.

Frequently Asked Questions

Q. *"When my daughter, Susan, plays on her tummy, she always uses her left hand. Her therapist wants me to encourage her to also play with her right hand. But, whenever Susan tries to reach with that hand, she rolls to the side. Why does this happen and what can I do to help her with this?"*

A. Although Susan plays well with her left hand, her left upper arm and shoulder muscles are weak. When Susan tries to reach with her right hand, the weight of her upper body is over her left elbow and forearm. If her arm muscles are not strong and coordinated enough, the elbow straightens, causing Susan to roll over onto her side.

Daily practice of *Tummy Time with Reach* will be helpful. When you do the exercise with Susan always have her reach with her right hand and support her upper left arm as much as needed. Stabilizing the left elbow by propping a small sandbag against it may be another way of preventing Susan from rolling to her side as she reaches. Or it may help if Susan's chest is propped on a roll-up towel as shown in activity *Independent Tummy Time Cradling Toys*.

Before you proceed talk to Susan's therapist about it and follow her recommendation.

Q. *"My son, Al, can prop himself up on big arms, but does not prop himself up on forearms and cannot play while lying on his tummy. Why is this so and what should I do?"*

A. Some children with cerebral palsy show an abnormal reflex pattern in stomach-lying or in a forward leaning position. When they lift their head or tilt it backwards, both of their arms stiffly stretch out forward; when they lower their head, both arms bend, are drawn to their chest, and may get stuck under their body. Al seems to show this reflex when he props up on his extended arms. He does not have the control of a child who pushes onto big arms. He cannot move his arms to the side, shift his weight, and briefly lift one arm. He is using all his arm muscles at once just to remain up on big arms.

Al has to learn to bend and straighten his elbows without moving his head at the same time. He needs to learn to reach with one arm and with both arms. Most likely he can learn this best in side-lying or supported sitting. Daily practice of "Shoulder-Elbow-Hand," "Rocking on Forearms," and "'Rocking and Reach" may benefit Al. But, do not start on your own. Work with Al's therapist. She or he knows Al. You will be most effective as a team.

Q. *"Missy is four years old and still not comfortable on her tummy. My husband and I believe this will not change and see no point in doing exercises in stomach lying. Missy's physical therapist still recommends them. Why?"*

A. Both you and the therapist have a valid point. If Missy does not like to be on her tummy by now, she probably never will be able to play on her tummy on her own. Nevertheless, if Missy doesn't mind being placed on her tummy if she is propped on a wedge or assisted by you, a daily play period in this position will be very beneficial for her. It will strengthen her back, neck, shoulder, and arm muscles. Strengthening these muscles will help her to sit up better and acquire the manual skills she still needs to learn.

Q. *"I am a special education preschool teacher. I think one of my students may benefit from several exercises in this chapter. Should I tell the school physical or occupational therapist about them?"*

A. Yes. I am sure the therapist will be glad about your initiative. Together, plan a good time for the therapist to show you how to work with your student.

Q. *"I feel uneasy about this. I am not trained to do therapy. Wouldn't it be better if the therapist did the exercises?"*

A. No. These are simple exercises. Feel free to do them as the child's therapist recommends them and teaches them to you. It is much better if you do them once or twice daily than if the therapist does them once a week.

Q. *"But these are home instructions. Wouldn't I interfere with what the parents do at home?"*

A. I am glad you bring this up. Yes, the parent should know about the exercises your student does during the school day. Most likely they will be very appreciative.

9

Guarding Against Falls

Children acquire basic motor skills during their first year of life. When infants first stand and walk, they learn by trial and error. They frequently lose their balance and fall. Fortunately, most of the time children can catch themselves with outstretched arms and do not get hurt. Children are not born with the capability to catch themselves when falling. It is an automatic response that emerges between four and twelve months of age.

The ability to quickly stretch out your arms to protect yourself from serious injury is called the *protective extension reaction.* When you lower six-month-old babies head first to the floor (mimicking a fall), their arms stretch out. They are ready to catch themselves. Do the same with three-month-old infants, and no response is seen.

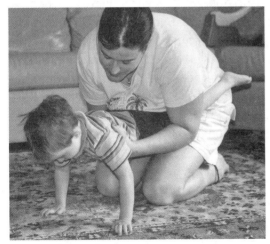

In sitting, infants can catch themselves when they fall forward at six months, to the sides by six to eight months, and backward by twelve months.

The protective extension reaction is an automatic response. This means that no voluntary effort is required. The situation—the danger of falling— triggers the response. Once established, the protective extension reaction will stay with you for the rest of your life. Test yourself. Sit or kneel on the floor and have another person push you in any direction. Notice how your body and your arms react.

Automatic reactions are faster than voluntary movements. From the time a person wants to move (voluntarily), it takes 200 milliseconds or more until he actually moves. For an automatic

9.1

reaction, this lag time (latency) is only 90 to 150 milliseconds. Speed is of the essence if you are falling. To protect you, your arms have to be faster than the force of gravity on your body.

The most crucial protective extension reaction is the one that protects us when we fall forward. It is often referred to as the ***parachute response*** because of the way it looks when children catch themselves with outstretched arms (photo 9.1). Children with spastic arm muscles who cannot straighten their arms or bear weight with them do not show a parachute response. The same is true for children with severe hypotonia whose arms are too weak for bearing weight. Most children who fail to develop an effective parachute response do not progress to independent walking without use of an assistive device such as a walker or crutches (Bleck, 1975).

Sometimes there appears to be an additional sensory component such as an aversion to touch or to weight bearing which the child needs to overcome before the parachute response emerges. The following story describes this.

The Boy Who Did Not Want to Touch the Floor

Ben, age one, came to therapy with both parents. He was small for his age, had big chubby cheeks, and a cute smile. Developmental gross motor testing showed that Ben had the skills of a five-month-old. He rolled, reached for toys, and played with them in back-lying. He did not like to be on his tummy and rolled out of this position quickly. Placed in a sitting position, he could hold his trunk nice and straight, yet within thirty seconds he would topple over to the side or backwards. Ben behaved just like many four- or five-month-old babies do.

There was a difference, however, when the therapist lowered Ben headfirst—he did not stretch out his arms to touch the floor, but drew them to his chest. Playing on his back, he stretched out his arms effortlessly. Why not in the other situation? Next the therapist tried to place him on hands and knees. His body and his muscles seemed to be ready for it. Yet, as soon as his hands touched the floor and his arms carried the weight of his upper body, he cried and tried to pull his arms to his chest as if in pain. Lowered to the floor feet first, Ben pulled his legs up and would not stand. When he was placed into standing with his legs supported, he cried and tried to pull his legs up as if he had been forced to stand on needles.

Why did Ben show these reactions? We do not know for sure. There are theories about these avoidance responses, but no conclusive facts. Ben may have a defect to the part of the brain that interprets information from the senses of touch or position. We do know, however, that if the parachute reaction does not emerge, the child most likely will learn to sit up but will not crawl on hands and knees, pull to stand, or walk.

Ben is only a year old. At this young age, treatment can still be effective. With therapy sessions and a home program, Ben can slowly learn to tolerate bearing weight on his arms and progress with his motor development. Is a good outcome certain? Unfortunately not.

Most physical therapists who work in pediatrics have encountered some children who avoid weight bearing. Your therapist will address the issue one week at a time, one therapy session at a time.

Right now, Ben has to get used to being on his tummy, as well as bearing weight on straight arms. Lots of tummy time is needed so that Ben has the opportunity to catch up, gain strength and coordination of his back and shoulder muscles, and start propping himself up on his forearms. Ben also has to practice weight bearing on his straight arms for very short time periods while sitting on the floor.

Ben detested both activities and let everyone know it. What to do? During therapy time, two motivated adults entertaining and fussing over him and a truly large toy closet made things more tolerable. Tummy time slowly but surely improved. Once Ben was able to hold his head up and look around, he realized that tummy time was not so bad after all.

Unfortunately, at home and at daycare, progress was not as easy. It was asking a great deal of daycare workers to do the extra work of placing one of their charges on his tummy and keeping him from crying. For a parent coming home from work, it would also be too much. Yet, the parents made a very sensible decision. Every time they put Ben down, they would place him on his tummy. Usually he did not stay long before he flipped over onto his back. He always did some playing, though, and best of all, he stopped crying about it. When his parents had time to relax on the floor with Ben, they would play with him and try to increase the amount of time he would stay on his tummy. This approach worked well. The parents observed that on his own Ben started to stay on his tummy for longer periods of time. The really good news came when Ben's mother beamed: "He likes to be on his tummy now. Last night he rolled onto it on his own."

How was sitting with arms propped coming along? Ben did not like to touch the floor with his hands—period. In sitting, he learned to straighten his back and lift his hands off the floor. So now, when Ben was placed with his arms propped, he did not mind. He just sat up and lifted his hands off the floor. The therapist then had Ben lean forward and again placed his hands firmly on the floor. Again he sat up straight. Ben could do five repetitions of these "touchdowns." So his new home instructions were to do five touchdowns. Ben's parents did them, and even the daycare workers found time to do the exercise with him.

During treatment sessions the therapist had been working on eliciting the parachute reaction. Ben showed progress. He no longer drew his arms to his chest. At times he would touch the surface lightly with one hand. It was a beginning.

Ben's progress in stomach-lying continued. He played on his tummy, he could move sideways, and he started to move backwards. Then one day it happened. Ben pushed himself up, his chest rose off the floor, and his arms stretched out with his hands firmly planted on the floor. Hooray, this was the breakthrough! He was no longer "the boy who did not want to touch the floor."

A couple of weeks later when the parachute reaction was practiced, Ben brought both arms forward. Both hands touched the surface. They landed lightly. More repetitions, and his hands came out faster and touched firmly. Soon it was fun. Instead of crying, he laughed as he bounced hands first off a softly inflated therapy ball.

Ben had become able to weight bear on his arms and acquired the parachute response in spite of his sensory problems. Weight bearing on feet was trained similarly and Ben started to tolerate it for short periods of time. Sometime later his sitting balance improved, he sat up by himself, and he started to crawl on hands and knees. Still, despite all his progress, Ben's sensory problems are persisting. More training will be needed before Ben will walk.

Encouraging Protective Extension Reaction Forward

The story of Ben shows how the parachute response can become effective after a child has learned to bear weight on his arms with straight elbows. Strong back, shoulder, and arm muscles are needed for this. Plenty of tummy time and early training of weight bearing on big arms made it happen for Ben.

For an effective protective extension reaction, children have to be able to bear weight on their arms without the elbows collapsing, and they have to be able to do so very quickly. If you fall forward on your arms and your elbows give out, your face will hit the floor—ouch! If you fall and your arms stretch out too slowly, you will get hurt too.

The subsequent activities encourage the development of the parachute response. Use them as directed by your child's therapist and follow any specific instructions given.

Touchdown in Sitting

1. Your child sits with arms propped.
2. You sit or kneel in front of him and put your hands around both elbows. Lift your child's arms slightly off the floor (photo 9.2a), pause, and then place them quickly down (photo 9.2b).
3. Next lift your child's arms a couple inches off the floor, pause, and then let them drop down.
4. When he is used to the exercise, lift his arms a little higher and then let them touch down.

Repeat 10 times.

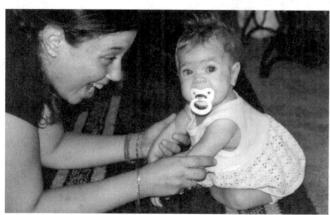

9.2a

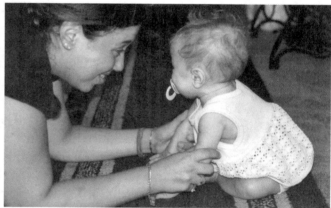

9.2b

Note: If your child fists or turns his hands so the back of the hand touches the floor, see if lifting the arms less will prevent this. If not, don't use the exercise. Your therapist can recommend an activity better suited for your child.

Flying Touchdown

1. While you are kneeling on the floor, hold your child facing away from you as shown in photo 9.3a. Support his chest with both hands. Your child's legs are hugging your waist.
2. Lower your child until his hands touch the floor (photo 9.3b). Then lift him up and repeat.

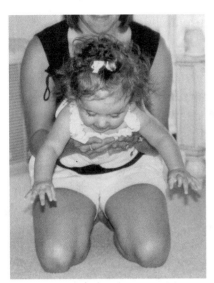
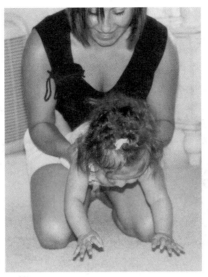
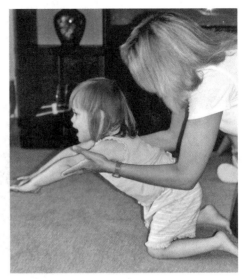

9.3a   9.3b   9.4

Keep your back straight so you do not strain it. Your child may like the activity but do not use it if it is too hard on your body.

Touchdown from Short Kneel

So far, you have practiced the protective reaction in easy situations. As your child masters these, he is ready for more taxing exercises that will firm up his skill and prepare him for everyday life situations. The development of the skill will give him the confidence that he needs to cope with unexpected balance loss.

This exercise is for children who can stay on hands and knees with little help but cannot yet balance in short kneel (kneeling with hips bent). Practice it on a carpeted floor.

1. Help your child to raise himself from hands and knees to short kneel by supporting him around the chest.
2. Tell him: "Stretch your arms out and put them on the floor," as you lower him. If needed, guide his arms forward as shown in photo 9.4.

Repeat 10 times.

After a good practice session, see if he will catch himself without your help. Warn him: "Be ready—put your arms out," as you take away your support and let him drop from short kneel onto his arms.

You want your child to become very good with touchdowns, so don't stop practicing as soon as he can do them. Practice 5 to 10 touchdowns daily for weeks, even months. The more you practice, the quicker and surer the arms will come forward. As your child becomes confident about catching himself, he will like the exercise. Now you may do the touchdowns as a reward after doing the more "boring" exercises like stretches.

Touchdown from Tall Kneel

When your child is able to short kneel, play in this position, and easily move out of it, he is ready for something more challenging. This "touchdown" exercise is for children who can tall kneel (kneeling with hips straight) at furniture.

1. Practice on a carpeted floor. Help your child to come to tall kneel and support him at his hips or around his chest (photo 9.5a).

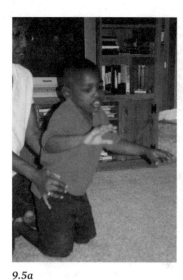

9.5a

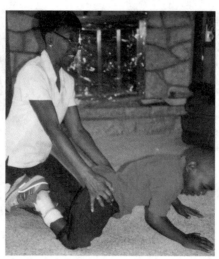

9.5b

2. Have him lean slightly forward and warn him: "r-e-a-d-y a-n-d touchdown," as you help him come down (photo 9.5b).

Repeat 10 times.

When your child can handle it, hold him at his hips or have him do the touchdowns on his own. Do daily practice sessions until the touchdowns are very well learned.

Note: In daily life, children (or adults) do not drop out of tall kneel this way. Instead, they lower themselves from tall kneel to short kneel, and then come to hands and knees or sit down. However, touchdowns from tall kneel will improve and perfect your child's protective extension reaction.

Encouraging Protective Extension Reaction to the Sides

SPECIAL PRACTICE FOR CHILDREN WITH HEMIPLEGIA

Protective extension reactions to the sides are important when children first sit and play in sitting. Their balance reactions are not yet refined and they easily topple over to the side. A stretched-out arm will save them, or at least break the fall. Later, when children begin to stand and walk, the protective extension reaction to the side will protect them from hurting their head if they fall sideways.

Children with good protective extension reactions in forward fall may acquire the ones to the sides with little training. Children with unequal arm skills, especially children with hemiplegia, however, need special training. Children with right hemiplegia will develop protective reactions forward and to the sides with their left arm, but need special training to acquire them with their right arm. Children with left hemiplegia will need training for left protective extension.

If your child has hemiplegia, your child's therapist may want you to start weight bearing exercises with your child's affected arm as early as possible. Early training is more effective and accomplishes more in a shorter time. It gives the affected arm a head start and prevents your child from neglecting that arm. It is also easier for you. A baby likes to sit with your support. He may not mind leaning on his affected arm as long as you give him the assistance he needs. A toddler, however, may have a definite opinion about things.

Use the exercises as directed by the therapist and closely follow any specific instructions given.

Weight Bearing on Straight Arm in Side Sitting

1. Sit on the floor with your child sitting between your legs facing away from you.
2. Place your open left hand against the inner side of your child's upper right arm. Use your fingers to straighten out his elbow.

3. With your other hand, open his right hand and place it on the floor.
4. After your child is in a good side leaning position, support his right elbow with your right hand. Place a toy in easy reach and have him play with his left hand.
5. Encourage your child to play in this position for two minutes, or as long as he likes. Support him less if he does well.

Reverse sides for practice with the left arm.

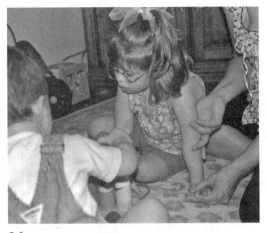

9.6

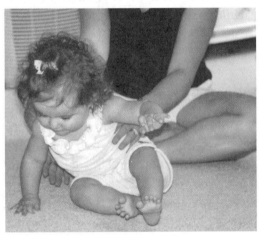

9.7

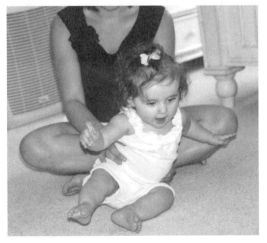

9.8

Variation A. If your child fists his hand, try this maneuver: Slide your open right hand around his wrist into his palm and open his hand. Place the back of your open hand on the floor so your child leans onto your hand with his open hand (photo 9.6). Have him side sit like this. If his hand stays open, slide your hand out from under his, placing his hand on the floor.

Variation B. If your child's arm is very weak or very spastic, your therapist may recommend that he wear a soft arm splint during the activity.

Note: Do not expect quick progress with this activity. Most likely it will take over a month of daily practice.

One Arm Touchdown to the Side

After children can support themselves sideways on one arm, they are ready for the next two exercises. Do them as directed by your child's therapist and follow any specific instructions given.

1. Your child sits facing away from you.
2. Hold him by the upper arms and move him toward the right side, guiding him to touch down with his right arm.

Repeat 10 times.

When your child does this well, give less guidance to the right arm and do the side movement faster (photo 9.7). Switch sides if you want to train the left arm.

Alternate Touchdown to the Sides

1. Hold your child around his chest.
2. Tip him to the right and then to the left for a touchdown (photo 9.8).
3. Play music or sing "I'm a little teapot…" for rhythm and fun.

Do 10 touchdowns alternating to the right and left side.

Note: If your child does well on one side but has difficulties on the other, do this exercise only occasionally. For daily practice, you may want to work with the less skilled arm as described for the "One-Arm Touchdown to the Side" exercise.

Frequently Asked Questions

Q. *"My daughter, Anna, is just learning to catch herself with her arms. She often has one hand fisted when I practice with her. I am worried that she is acquiring a bad habit. Shouldn't both her hands be open?"*

A. First let her do it however she can and worry about perfection later. Most likely the fisting will slowly but surely diminish.

At the same time, you have a valid point about not teaching a bad habit. Share your thoughts with Anna's physical therapist. Knowing Anna, she will be able to give you good advice.

Q. *"Our daughter Liana does not like to touch things. Her occupational therapist says she is sensory defensive and has problems with sensory integration. She showed me how to brush Liana to reduce her sensitivity. Why didn't you recommend brushing?"*

A. This book is about teaching motor skills. It shows how children like Liana and Ben can learn basic motor skills. If your child has significant problems with sensory processing, it is wise to work with an occupational therapist with training in these issues.

Q. *"My son, Rick, has hemiplegia. His right arm is very weak and uncoordinated. His therapist gave me home instructions to practice side sitting and leaning on his right arm. I have to support his right elbow and shoulder while he sits this way. Rick doesn't mind it because I let him play with his Matchbox cars, which he loves. But I am frustrated. Rick's arm does not seem to get any better. What should I do?"*

A. The activity the therapist gave you is very good. It will train Rick to bear weight with his right arm. This is very useful and will make his arm stronger as well as more coordinated. Using his favorite toys during the exercise is fun for Rick. Just hang in there, do the exercise daily, and your efforts will pay off. Yes, progress may be very slow. It may feel like you are sitting on your lawn watching the grass grow. Share your frustrations with Rick's therapist. Together you can find a solution. The therapist may recommend bracing the right arm with a soft elbow splint. The splint may provide enough support that Rick could side sit without your help. This will make exercise time easier for both of you. Also, it is my experience that progress is easier to see and to judge when you are not involved in supporting the child.

10

Sitting Pretty

Meet Elli

Elli is sitting up! Elli's parents are happy and proud, with good reason. Sitting is a major milestone in the gross motor development of any baby. As infants develop, they typically learn to sit up without support between six and eight months. Children with cerebral palsy need more time. The physical therapist's objective is to have them sit up by the time they are two years old. This is because children with cerebral palsy who sit by two years of age are more likely to walk than children who have not achieved this goal. Sitting by two is a major treatment goal and therapists want their little patients to sit with a nice straight back. They want them to sit pretty.

Elli is eleven and a half months old. She was referred to therapy because her physician was worried about her gross motor development. At the time of her doctor's visit two weeks ago, Elli still wasn't able to sit on her own. As mom brings Elli to therapy, she wonders: "Because Elli is able to sit now, maybe she does not need physical therapy after all."

The assessment shows that Elli sits with poor balance and posture. Her back is rounded, and her shoulders and head are hunched forward. Instead of resting on the floor, her knees stick up. Falling backwards is Elli's way of getting herself out of sitting. Once on the floor, she needs help to sit back up. Elli is not able to crawl or pull to stand.

The therapist supports the physician's recommendation that Elli will benefit from physical therapy. The parents agree and weekly treatment is started. The therapist concentrates on strengthening the trunk muscles, especially back muscles. She trains

Elli's sitting balance and all missing age-appropriate gross motor skills. The parents work with Elli at home, following the therapist's instructions.

After six months, Elli is showing good progress. She is able to move in and out of sitting on her own, come up onto her hands and knees, and crawl. She enjoys crawling everywhere. Standing is still difficult, however. Her trunk leans forward against the table in front. If the therapist or her parents do not help, her legs turn in and her heels rise off the floor.

How is Elli sitting? Her back is stronger, and her sitting balance has improved. She sits nice and straight on a little stool or the therapy ball. On the floor, however, Elli does not sit pretty at all. As before, her back is rounded, and because her legs have grown, her knees stick up even higher off the floor.

Why has Elli made no progress with sitting on the floor? It has to do with the position of the hipbone (pelvis). **When we sit straight, our pelvis is in an upright (neutral) position; it is neither tilted forward nor backward**. Sitting straight requires coordinated work of low back, hip, and low stomach muscles. Maintaining a good sitting posture is difficult for children with cerebral palsy, and it is even harder to sit on the floor than on a chair.

Find this out for yourself. Sit straight in a chair with your hands on your hips. Tip your pelvis forward (your low back arches), tip it backwards (your low back rounds), and then hold that in-between position with your back straight. Notice how it feels. Next, sit on the floor with your legs out in front of you and your hands on your hips. Do you notice that your hips want to tip backwards, rounding your back? It takes effort to bring your pelvis into an upright position and sit tall and straight. This happens because your hamstring muscles are stretched and pull your pelvis backwards when you sit on the floor. When you sit in a chair with knees bent, your hamstrings are not stretched and do not pull your pelvis backward. Therefore, it is easier to keep the pelvis upright and sit nice and straight.

Elli has gained the strength and coordination to hold her pelvis upright when she sits in a chair, but not enough to do so on the floor. Elli's hamstring muscles are tight, which makes floor sitting especially difficult for her. When Elli plays on the floor, she seldom sits with her legs in front. She prefers to crawl or kneel. In kneeling, she likes to rest her bottom on her heels—a position which therapists call heel sitting or short kneeling. This is her favorite play position.

During the following year of therapy, Elli masters many more skills and she starts to walk on her own. She does not have a good walking pattern; one foot turns in and she often toe walks with the other foot. Yet, Elli gets around and that's what matters. Floor sitting has improved just a little over the year.

Realizing how difficult the floor sitting position is for Elli, the therapist has decided that Elli needs some extra help. When she works with Elli on the floor, she has her sit with legs spread apart, her knees slightly bent and turned out. She helps Elli to sit straight and then drapes two five-pound ankle weights or sandbags over each thigh. The weight of the bags helps ground her legs to the floor. This gives her a wide base of support and makes it easier for Elli to keep her trunk straight. She no longer has to hunch her shoulders and bend forward to stay seated.

Floor sitting is important for small children. It stretches the hamstring muscles, and stretches and strengthens the muscles around the hip joint; the muscles of the low back, stomach, and thigh work together in a coordinated way. Sitting with legs apart and turned out puts healthy pressure into the hip joint and helps the growing joint form a nice socket for the head of the upper leg bone (femur) to nestle in.

At home Elli sits with her sandbags for half an hour each day when she watches her favorite TV show. In preschool she uses the bags during story time. She does not mind using them because this way she does not have to sit in a chair but can join her friends on the floor sitting pretty.

Helping Your Child to Sit

Elli's story is typical of children with diplegia. The muscle tone of the legs is increased and the back and stomach muscles usually are very weak. Children with quadriplegia have similar problems. They too need help with sitting.

In order to sit on the floor, children need:

- *Strong trunk muscles.* Strong back and stomach muscles will hold your child's trunk up while sitting. When you work with your child while in a stomach- or back-lying position, you strengthen her trunk muscles. This gets her ready to sit.
- *Balance.* Pure strength is not enough. For the children to develop trunk control and balance their muscles have to work together in a coordinated way. When your child sits with a straight back and as little support as possible, her balance will be challenged. With experience, her balance responses will improve.
- *Flexible hamstring muscles.* Hamstrings that are too short pull the pelvis backwards and make it next to impossible for your child to sit on the floor like other children. Doing daily straight leg stretches with your child will keep the hamstring muscles flexible. (See Chapter 5.)

Supported Sitting

Before your child can sit by herself, you need to support her. Your child's physical therapist will show you how to place and support your child in a good, straight sitting position. Your child's first accomplishment will be to hold her head up in supported sitting. Next the therapist will guide you to lower your level of support and challenge your child to hold her head and upper trunk up by herself. The more progress your child makes, the lower you will place your hands as you support her. Finally, you will need to support her just at her hips.

The following are examples of how to support your child in sitting. Use them as directed by your child's therapist and follow any specific instructions she may give you.

Sitting with Chest Support
1. Sit on the floor with your legs apart and have a toy ready for play.
2. Place your child sideways between your legs. Her legs are apart, turned out and slightly bent at the knee.

3. Support your child with your left open flat hand against her lower back and your right open hand flat against her chest. Give firm pressure with your hands so she sits straight and tall.

4. Next help her bend from the hip so her trunk tilts forward. You want her to lean forward into your right hand support or against your right leg (whichever works best and is most comfortable for you) while keeping her back straight.

5. Encourage your child to play with a toy in front (photo 10.1).

Variation. After your child is used to the position, see if she is able to keep her back straight without your supportive hand at her lower back. If she can, turn her so she faces away from you and support only her chest with your open flat hand (photo 10.2).

Keep watching your child's lower back. If she slouches backward, intermittently give lower back support and correct her posture. Do not have your child lean back and rest against you.

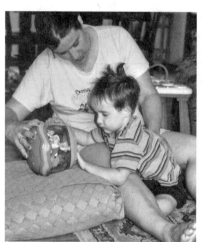 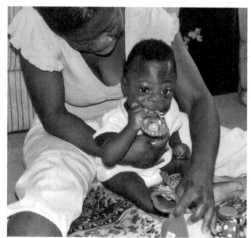 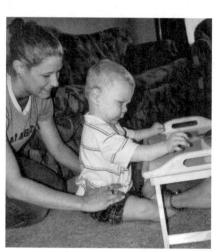

10.1   10.2   10.3

Sitting with Hip Support at a Table

After your child is able to hold her trunk nice and straight with chest support, she may be ready to sit with low back or hip support.

Equipment. For this activity you need a low bench or table. A bed tray would make a good table for a small child. A taller child may sit better at a low bench or a step stool. A low coffee table may be best for an older child.

1. Place your child in front of the table with her legs apart, turned out, and slightly bent at the knee.

2. From the side, support her firmly with one hand against her lower back and the other hand against her chest. Have her sit straight and tall.

3. Help her lean forward and place her arms on the table.

4. Take your chest support away and only support her low back while your child leans on her arms or against the table and plays.

Variation. Sit or kneel behind your child. Open your hands wide and firmly hold her hips from the sides between your thumbs and fingers. This way you will be able to keep her low back and trunk straight or slightly tilted forward (photo 10.3). Encourage her to lean with her arms on the table and play with a toy in front of her.

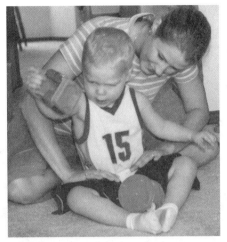

10.4

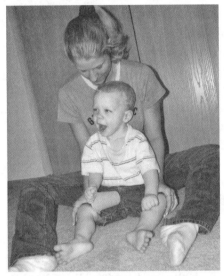

10.5

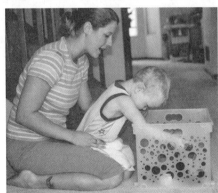

10.6

Sitting with Hip Support

1. Sit or kneel on the floor.
2. Your child sits between your legs facing away from you. Your child's legs are apart, turned out, and slightly bent at the knee.
3. Open your hands wide and firmly hold her hips from the sides between your thumbs and fingers. With the little finger side of your hand give some downward pressure to her thighs (photo 10.4).
4. You want your child to sit with a straight back, tilting slightly forward.
5. Encourage her to play with a toy in front of her.

Sitting with Thigh Support

After your child sits well with hip support:

1. Move your hands from her hips and place them firmly on her upper thighs close to her groin.
2. See if your child does well with the reduced support (photo 10.5).
3. Increase your support whenever your child starts to slouch backward.

Do not have your child lean back and rest against you. Keep her interested in playing with the toys in front her. If she gets tired, encourage her to lean more forward and support herself with her arms propped on the floor or have her take a rest snuggling in your lap.

Heel Sitting with Hip Support at a Crate

A child who sits well with hip support most likely will enjoy the next activity in heel sitting (also called short kneeling) at a crate. This position allows her to be up higher and brings variety into her sitting routine.

1. Heel sit on the floor and help your child to sit the same way wedged between your thighs (photo 10.6).
2. Have a plastic crate with interesting things inside in front of your child. Encourage her to hold onto the rim of the crate with her left hand.
3. Place your hand over hers to secure it. With your other hand, support your child at the hip.
4. Encourage her to play with her right hand.

Do not allow your child to lean with her chest against the crate and play with both hands. If she gets tired holding on with her left hand, have her switch hands—then hold on with her right and play with her left hand. Learning to always hold on with one hand will make her independent sooner.

Independent Sitting with Arm Support

After your child is able to sit well with hip or thigh support, you may expect that she will start sitting without any support. Unfortunately, this may not happen soon. Many children with cerebral palsy make good progress with supported sitting and then, when they seem ready to sit on their own, progress stalls. Why does this happen? It has to do with the nature of cerebral palsy. Gaining the strength to hold up the trunk is easier to achieve for the children than developing good coordination and sufficient balance.

Sitting on the floor is especially difficult for most children. When sitting without support, spastic and tight inner thigh and hamstring muscles affect their posture and interfere with emerging balance reactions. You can reduce the influence of these muscles if you have your child sit with her bottom on a folded beach towel. Now the hips are higher than the legs, less bending occurs at the hips, the hamstrings are less stretched, and therefore the backwards pull of the pelvis diminishes. Placing weights over your child's thighs will further improve her stability.

Yet, even when you place your child on a towel and use weights to stabilize her legs, she may not have enough balance to sit on her own. Unsupported, she may stay up for only a few seconds and then topple over.

What can you do to help her? Supporting her in sitting for hours each day will become old quickly and may not even help. Your child may get used to your support and rely on it. You may place your child in a special chair with good support. She will sit well and play well in the chair, yet her balance will not be challenged and, therefore, will not improve. For her balance to improve further, your child needs to sit on her own and support herself with her arms.

When children sit quietly with arm support, they experience how gravity affects them. Slowly, they may learn what they need to do to stay up. First, they sit leaning forward supporting themselves with both arms all the time. The more they sit this way, the longer they can do it. Next they will sit up straighter, dare to lift one or both hands off the support, and sit free for short periods. ***Quiet play will help them stay up longer.*** Later, after their balance has improved, they may dare to do larger arm or body movements without toppling over.

The following examples demonstrate ways to place your child so that she can support herself with her arms all by herself. Have your child's therapist help you choose a position and practice it with your child. Follow the therapist's specific instructions when you practice with your child at home.

Sitting with Propped Arms

1. Your child's legs are apart, turned out, and slightly bent at the knee.
2. Help her to bend at her hips, lean forward, and place both hands on the floor (photo 10.7).
3. If it is difficult for your child to sit this way—her back is rounded and her knees do not rest on the floor—have her sit on a folded-up beach towel and place a five-pound ankle weight or sandbag over each thigh to weigh them down and stabilize them. (See the Appendix for instructions on making the sandbag.)

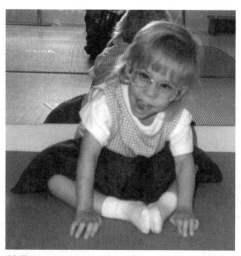

10.7

This is a very good position for children to learn to sit safely all by themselves. They have a wide base of support and they can use their arms to support them. Yet, children do not like to sit this way. To them it is rather pointless to sit and do nothing. With the hands planted on the floor, they can't even suck their thumb. Most children soon realize: "If I let myself fall to the side this exercise is over fast." So they don't try to stay up—unless, that is, you entertain your child while she sits. You might sing or show a picture book to a younger child, but to motivate an older child to sit this way is definitely harder.

One way to get around this is to embed the exercise into other activities. You know your child enjoys sitting and playing on the floor with your support. Next time you do this, give her just one toy to play with and set the rest aside. Now each time she wants a different toy, tell her to lean forward and place her hands on the floor and sit by herself, while you get the toy. Start out slowly by requiring her to sit by herself for only 2 to 5 seconds. If it works, go for 8 seconds the following week and so on.

Once your child is able to wait for you without losing her balance while you search for another toy in the next room, you know she has made good progress and acquired a very useful skill. From now on, you can sit her down this way for a short time whenever it is convenient for you without having to worry that she will fall to the side and hurt her head. You taught your child something that is of importance to both of you. What she learned by your persistent initiative brings her a big step closer to sitting and playing on her own. And there is a fringe benefit. Each time she sits with arms propped, her hamstrings are stretched as well—something that is very helpful indeed.

Sitting with Back Support and Play

The following activities show you how to position your child so she can sit and play on her own. They are popular home instructions, well liked by parents and children. They will give both of you some free time of your own. With the help of your child's therapist, choose the one best suited for your child and follow the therapist's specific directions.

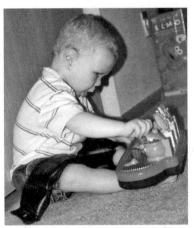

10.8a

1. Help your child to sit with good back support (against a wall, stair step, couch, or other solid piece of furniture).
2. Her legs are spread apart, turned out, and slightly bent at the knee. The hip is bent and the trunk leans slightly forward.
3. Drape a five-pound ankle weight or sandbag over each thigh for stability.
4. If your child's pelvis is tilted backwards, causing her back to round, wedge a rolled-up towel between the wall and her low back. It will also help if she sits on a folded-up beach towel. With her seat higher than her legs it will be easier for her to sit straight.
5. Place a sturdy toy in front of her or on her legs. Encourage her to lean forward and brace herself with one hand on the floor, on her legs, or on the toy while playing with her other hand (photo 10.8a). A busy box or a pop-up toy is a good toy to use.
6. If your child is in danger of falling to the sides, place pillows on each side.

Variation A. Some children do not sit well in this position. Their upper back and shoulders may hunch forward. It helps the children if the toy they play with is placed over their legs or propped up slightly slanted toward them.

Also, if your child cannot sit with her legs turned out and slightly bent at the knee, have her cross her legs and tailor sit (10.8b).

Variation B. Observe your child. If you feel she is no longer in danger of falling backwards, you may have her play without back support. For safety, place a big pillow behind her.

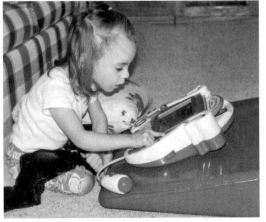

10.8b

Sitting with Arms Supported at a Table

Equipment. For this activity, you need a low bench or table. A bed tray would make a good table for a small child. A taller child may sit better at a low bench or stepping stool. A low coffee table may be best for an older child. Parents may also purchase an adjustable floor table.

1. Your child sits in front of the table with her legs placed under the table.
2. Her legs are apart, turned out, and slightly bent at the knee. If needed, stabilize the legs with weights as before.
3. Help her to sit straight, lean forward, and support herself with her arms on the table.
4. Place pillows at her sides and behind her to soften a possible fall or have her sit in front of a couch.
5. From her side or front, show her a picture book or read a story (photo 10.9a).
6. After your child can sit quietly with both arms propped, see if she can play with a toy that requires minimal arm movements (photo 10.9b). A busy box may work well with a younger child and an older child may enjoy paging through a book.

Variation. If your child quickly loses balance when playing, sit in front and stabilize her resting arm by firmly placing your open flat hand on her hand and forearm. Do this for the next one to three weeks and then have her try to play by herself.

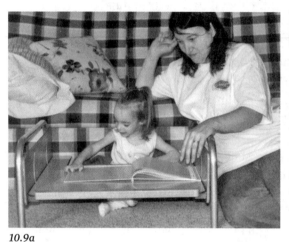
10.9a

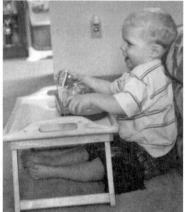
10.9b

Sitting without Arm Support

The more time children spend sitting on the floor in a good position—with the pelvis in neutral, the back straight, and leaning slightly forward—the more opportunity they have to improve their sitting balance. Instead of using their hands for support, they like to play with them. First they very briefly play with both hands and then brace themselves again with one hand on the floor, on their leg, or on the toy they play with. As they gain the confidence that they can hold themselves up with their trunk muscles, they gradually use their arms less for support. Sitting without arm support will challenge their balance responses. They slowly improve with practice.

The following activity recommendations are for children who sit on their own for short periods but cannot sit and play independently for a longer time. Use them if your therapist recommends it. The first one is especially helpful if your child tends to fall backwards. You have her sit between your legs facing you. This way your child has a forward orientation—she will more likely lean forward and catch herself with her arms if she loses her balance.

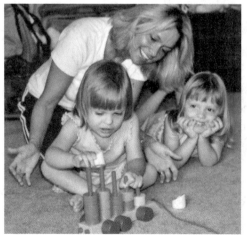
10.10

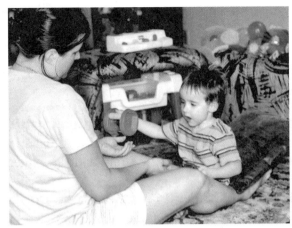

10.11

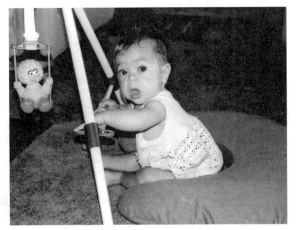

10.12

Sitting Between Your Legs

1. Sit with your legs stretched out and apart.
2. Your child sits between your legs, facing you, with a pillow behind her. Brace her with your legs.
3. Encourage her to play with a toy in front of her (photo 10.11).
4. As your child gains balance, move your legs a few inches apart challenging her to sit and play independently.
5. Watch her closely and be ready to give her support as needed.

Sitting at the Baby Gym

1. Have your child sit at the side of the baby gym.
2. Encourage her to hold onto the crossbar with one hand and play with the small toys mounted there with the other hand (photo 10.12). A baby gym is not sturdy but may provide the light support your child may still need.

For a small child, a Boppy pillow will be a good protection in the event of a side or backwards fall.

SUGGESTIONS FROM PARENTS

What else can you do to encourage your child to sit up longer? The next recommendations come from parents.

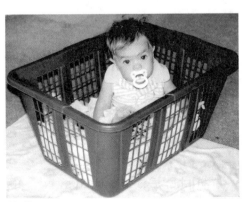

10.13

Have your child sit in a laundry basket.

"I have my daughter sit in the basket with the laundry that comes out of the dryer," says one mother. "She enjoys playing with the warm clothes when I sort the laundry."

A laundry basket with a non-slip mat at the bottom placed into your bathtub may also provide a secure space for your child to sit in during her bath (photo 10.13). It may allow her to play during bath time with your close supervision. It will *not be safe enough* to leave your child even momentarily by herself.

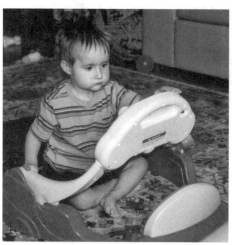

Have your child sit in the corner of the playpen or crib.

Sue reports: "Nick loves his playpen. I have him sit in a corner and put his favorite cars in front of him. In the playpen they can't roll far. He has gotten so good now, he can get the cars from even the furthest corner of the playpen."

Make a protected corner with couch cushions.

"I take the seat cushions off our couch and make a play area for Jason," Rose explains. "That's where he sits and plays when I get dinner."

Let Your Child Sit at a Play Station or Similar Toy.

"Sam tends to fall backwards when he sits and plays. With the entertainment and support in front of him he is less likely to do so," reports his mother (photo 10.14).

10.14

INDEPENDENT FLOOR SITTING

For many children with cerebral palsy, sitting on the floor with their legs out in front of them will never be easy. When they sit this way, their legs will not fully rest on the floor and they have a hard time sitting straight and maintaining their balance. Weighting their legs down helps them. As described in the story of Elli, floor sitting is important. It stretches and strengthens the muscles around the hip joint, and with the knees almost straight, it stretches the hamstring muscles. If the knees are more bent and turned out, the inner thigh muscles are stretched. All these stretches are good for your child.

In addition to using weights to help your child sit in this position, it may help if your child's hips are higher than her legs. This way the hamstrings are stretched less and the backwards pull to the pelvis is diminished. Again, follow specific recommendations your child's therapist gives you.

The Right Weights for Your Child. Your child's therapist will help you find the right weights for your child. Five-pound ankle weights draped over each thigh usually work well, but some children do better with heavier weights. Some parents like homemade sandbags best because they are softer and you can shift the sand and contour the bag to the leg. (See the Appendix for instructions on making sandbags.)

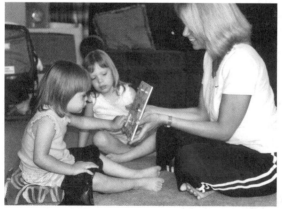
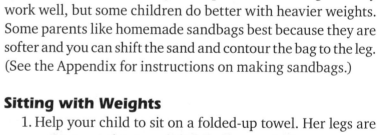
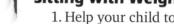

Sitting with Weights

1. Help your child to sit on a folded-up towel. Her legs are apart, turned out, and slightly bent at the knee.
2. Drape an ankle weight over each thigh for support.
3. Sit in front of her, encourage her to sit straight, bend at her hips, lean slightly forward, and play with you as long as she likes (photo 10.15).

10.15

Sitting with Weights during Independent Play

If your child does well sitting on a towel and with her legs stabilized by weights have her sit like this during independent playtime.

1. Place her favorite toy on, between, or in front of her legs (photo 10.16).
2. Let her play as long as she wants.
3. Give her a new toy when she is bored with the one she has.

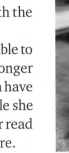

Variation. As soon as your child becomes able to crawl and move about on the floor, she will no longer like to sit still and play in one place. From now on have her sit with weights only when she sits still while she watches a video or TV, when you play with her or read a story, or during circle time in school or daycare.

Note: Do not have your child sit this way if she

10.16

leans to the side or straightens one leg at the knee and turns it inward.

ACTIVITIES FOR OLDER CHILDREN

As soon as your child can sit and play on the floor, have her do things for herself. It will further improve her balance and make her independent in small ways. The following suggestions are for children like Elli, who are two years or older and still need to improve their sitting balance.

Taking Off Socks—Pulling On Socks

The first job for your child to learn will be to take off her socks.

1. Start out by supporting her at her hips while she leans far forward to reach her feet. Give her time, let her struggle on her own, and try as hard as she can to pull her socks off (photo 10.17a).
2. As it becomes obvious that help is needed, push the socks partially over her heels and then let her try again. ***Regardless of how much you have to help initially, you always want her to do the last part all by herself*** (photo 10.17b).
3. Each week increase the part she does until she can take the socks off all on her own.

Now it will be her job to do this each night.

Work similarly with her to put on socks.

1. Start by putting the sock over her foot and then have her pull it up (photo 10.17c).
2. Next, put the sock just over her forefoot and have her do the rest. Increase what she does until she can put on her socks independently.

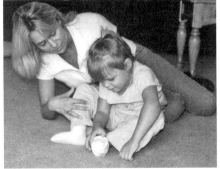

10.17a

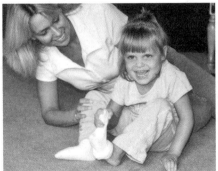

10.17b

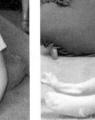

10.17c

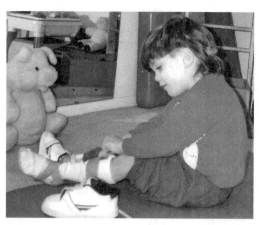
10.18

Taking Off Shoes and Braces

This is a two-part job.

1. First the laces or the Velcro have to be loosened; then the shoes or braces have to be removed (photo 10.18).
2. Work with your child as before. Give her plenty of time to work on her own. If help is needed, give it during the initial part, and always have her do the last part on her own.
3. Encourage your child to lift and draw up her foot when taking off the brace or shoe.
4. Once she can do it, it is your child's job to do it each night. It may take her five or more minutes in the beginning. Don't worry. Let her struggle—it will be time well spent.

Variation. If your child struggles to keep her balance when she sits on the floor, have her sit in a corner. Look for suitable corner places: in the kitchen between the refrigerator and wall, or a pulled out bottom drawer and the next cabinet, in the bathroom between the tub and wall, in the bedroom between the chest of drawers and the wall. It may give her the support she needs to become independent.

Other Ways to Sit on the Floor

HEEL SITTING

Elli was already walking but still struggled with sitting on the floor. Her story is not unusual for children with cerebral palsy. Most avoid sitting this way. Instead they choose to kneel and sit down on their heels. Their feet are bent down with toes pointing inwards and the heels turned out. Therapists call this heel sitting or short kneeling (photo 10.19).

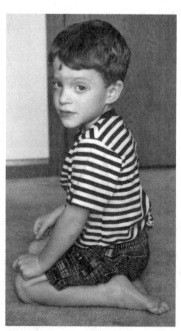
10.19

Why do the children like to sit this way? Let's find out. Kneel on the floor and lower yourself so your bottom rests on your heels. Place your hands on your hips and notice how easy it is to keep your pelvis forward and your back straight. Now stretch your legs out, sit on the floor, and do the same. You notice that your pelvis wants to drop backwards, rounding your lower back and making it harder to sit straight.

When sitting on their heels, it is easier for children to keep their pelvis upright, their trunk straight, and to balance. It makes using their hands and playing easier. This is why heel sitting is a very functional position for children with cerebral palsy.

The drawback of heel sitting is that the hips and knees are bent and the ankles are bent down. Children who always heel sit do not stretch out their hamstrings and calf muscles. Therefore, these muscles tend to become too short. If your child prefers to heel sit when she plays on her own, see to it that she sits with legs stretched out several times each day. Make it a habit that she sits this way when you play with her or read to her, or when she watches a video or TV. (If recommended by the therapist, have your child sit on a wedge or folded-up beach towel and place weights over her thighs.)

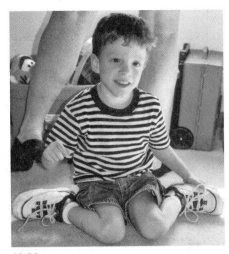 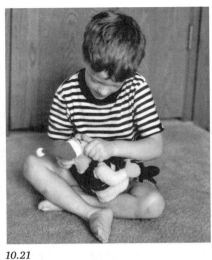 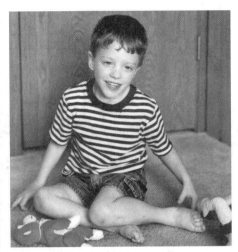

10.20   *10.21*   *10.22*

W-SITTING

When w-sitting, children turn their legs inwards, push their knees together, let the lower legs splay out to the sides, and sit on the floor between them (photo 10.20). The toes are pointing outwards. Similar to heel sitting, the position makes it easy to keep the pelvis upright, the trunk straight, and to balance. Because the lower legs are out to the side, enlarging the base of support, w-sitting is an extra stable position. No wonder that many children with cerebral palsy choose to sit this way. It allows them to play and use their hands well.

Unfortunately w-sitting has a negative effect. In this position the legs turn extremely inwards, which causes stress to the hip and knee joints. Therefore, long periods of w-sitting should be avoided. You may encourage your child to play also in side sitting, heel sitting, or tailor sitting. Yet, in all these positions, the child's legs are bent. Therefore, to keep her legs flexible, it is important for your child to sit several times a day with her legs stretched out. Follow the recommendations given above.

TAILOR SITTING

In this position, also known as "sitting cross-legged," the legs are bent and crossed in front (photo 10.21). It is a stable position that your therapist may recommend. It puts normal pressure into the hip joint and stretches the muscles of the inner thigh. For children with cerebral palsy it is easier to tailor sit than sit with legs stretched out in front of them. It is a good position for them when they sit for a longer period of time. Tailor sitting has the drawback that moving in or out of the position is difficult and many children need help with it.

Tailor sitting does not stretch the hamstring muscles as floor sitting with legs in front does. Therefore, parents are advised to use both positions with their children.

SIDE SITTING

When side sitting, a child sits mostly on one side with her legs bent toward the other side. Side sitting provides a large base of support (photo 10.22). It is a stable play position, especially if the child leans on one arm and plays with the other.

Your therapist may recommend side sitting for children with cerebral palsy. However, side sitting puts uneven pressure into the hip joints and your child may slump to the side instead of sitting straight. This position should not be used for long time periods, especially if your child strongly favors one side over the other.

Variability of Sitting

At one time or another, all children sit in every position mentioned above. They also sit with their legs placed out in front of them in a variety of ways. At times one leg may be straight while the other is bent at the knee. One leg may point forward one minute and be out to the side the next. Who likes to sit still in one spot? Not young children playing on the floor. They constantly move and change their position while pushing cars, building towers, or dressing dolls. In doing so, they use and stretch all their leg muscles at one time or another.

Children with cerebral palsy show less variety of positions when sitting. Most likely your child likes to play in heel sitting or tailor sitting. In both positions, her knees are always bent and her feet always point down. While sitting this way, she will not stretch her hamstrings and calf muscles or freely move her feet—unless you make it part of her daily routine. Telling your child, "No video or TV unless you sit with your legs out in front (and weights over the thighs if needed)" does not make you a mean parent. It makes you a caring parent! You are taking care that all muscles stay at optimal length. Daily sitting with sandbags and daily leg stretches will help ensure that when your child is ready to walk she has the flexibility to do so. This is something she cannot do for herself—and her therapist cannot do it alone either.

Sitting on a Bench or Chair

In western culture, adults prefer to sit on furniture. At work or at dinner we sit in a chair, on a bench, or on a stool. At leisure time we recline in a soft chair or sofa. When we travel we sit in a car, a plane, train, or on a bike or horse. Only preschool children like to sit and play on the floor most of the time. When children attend school, they too will spend more time sitting in chairs. Over a lifetime, sitting well on a chair rather than on the floor becomes an important skill.

We may sit in a chair a variety of ways. We may sit without back support—sitting straight or leaning forward. (Therapists call it bench sitting.) In these positions, our hands are free to do work. When we relax we sit differently. We lean backwards with our backs curving against the back of the chair. If the chair's backrest tilts backwards, we may lean back with a straight back—as we do when we unwind in a recliner.

Reclined sitting differs significantly from sitting straight up or forward leaning. In a reclined position our back muscles relax. If we do work in this position we mostly use the muscles in front of our body, similar to the way we use them when back-lying. On the other hand, sitting straight or leaning forward requires work of all trunk muscles, especially the back muscles, and it requires balance. The straighter our trunk is, the better our balance is, and the better we can use our hands.

Usually young children never sit in small chairs until after they are able to walk well. This is different for children with developmental delays or cerebral palsy. Recognizing how important a good sitting posture is, physical therapists start to work on bench sitting as early as possible. Especially for children who cannot sit well on the floor, training of good posture and balance will be done in bench sitting.

As mentioned before, sitting on a bench is easier for children with cerebral palsy than sitting on the floor. When sitting on a bench, the knees are bent, the hamstrings are not stretched, and short or spastic hamstring muscles will not pull the pelvis backwards. This makes it easier for children to sit with their trunk straight.

Unfortunately, chair sitting also poses problems for children with cerebral palsy. If they are just learning to sit on their own and have poor balance, sitting on a chair or bench is dangerous. A fall may seriously hurt them. Another problem is how they can safely get into or out of a chair on their own. Usually people sit down from standing and get up into standing. For children who are not able to stand, moving in and out of a chair is a big challenge.

When your therapist recommends that you work with your child in bench sitting, safety has to be a priority. Even when your child sits well without any support, stay next to her and *do not* walk away even momentarily. Only when she is able to stand up or get down from the bench on her own consistently will she be ready to sit without being guarded. At that time she may enjoy sitting in a child-size chair at a play table and looking at books, coloring, etc.

The following are examples of activities or exercises, which help to improve your child's sitting posture and balance. Use them as recommended by your child's therapist.

Equipment. For these sitting exercises, you need a good seat for your child. It needs to be of the right height for your child's feet to rest comfortably on the floor and preferably have a nonskid surface. Step stools have such a surface, come in various sizes, and are inexpensive. Use a stool just the right size for your child. A small child may also sit on a twelve-pack of soft drinks and an older child may sit on an upside down plastic crate. Some parents may decide to buy an adjustable therapy bench for their child. They are comfortably padded and wide enough so older children may place their arms at the side for support, and the seat height can be adjusted as the children grow.

Some parents have discovered that the first step of their stairs is just the right height for their child and use it for her sitting balance training. If the height of your step is such that your child's knees are bent about 90 degrees when her feet are on the floor, you may find it convenient to use.

Early Bench Sitting with Hip Support

1. Have your child sit on a stool placed in front of a couch or on the first step of your stairs (if of the right height).
2. Kneel in front of your child.
3. Have her lean against the back support while you place her legs in a good position. You want her knees bent, slightly apart, and her feet flat on the floor pointing forward.

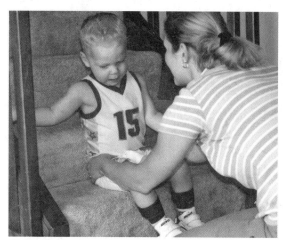

10.23

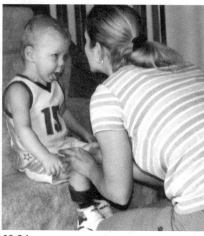

10.24

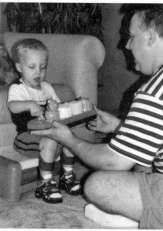

10.25

4. Next, place your wide-open hands at the side of her hips, with your thumbs in front and your fingers in the back. Tip her pelvis upwards, so her lower back is straight and encourage her to sit straight (photo 10.23). With her pelvis stabilized in a good position she may be able to sit tall. If she does:

5. Hold her for a couple of minutes while you sing a song or talk to her.

Early Bench Sitting with Leg Support

1. Follow the directions for Early Bench Sitting with Hip Support, above.
2. After you child sits well with your help, move your hands away from her hips, place them on her thighs or knees, and give light downward pressure.
3. Encourage her to sit tall while you talk or sing a song together (photo 10.24).

Variation. If your child cannot sit straight—her pelvis tips backwards and her lower back slouches—see if it helps her if you wedge a piece of foam or a rolled-up towel between her lower back and the back support.

Bench Sitting with Play

After your child can sit still with minimal support from you, she may enjoy playing with a toy you hold up for her.

1. Your child sits on a stool placed in front of a couch.
2. Help her to sit tall with feet flat on the floor and knees apart.
3. Kneel or sit in front of her and hold up a sturdy toy for her to play with (photo 10.25).

While playing, she may lose her good posture. If this happens, try to correct her without interrupting her play. If this is not possible, place the toy temporarily to the side, and ask her to sit tall with your help.

Sitting and Reaching

1. Your child sits on a stool placed in front of a couch.
2. Help her to sit tall with feet flat on the floor and knees apart.
3. Kneel or sit in front of her.
4. Hold up small toys and have her reach for them. Hold them in easy reach (photo 10.26). You want to make sure she can control her arm movements without losing her good sitting balance.

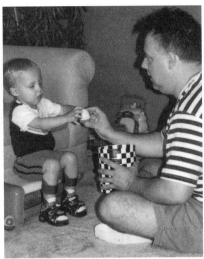
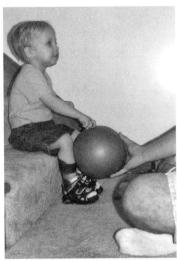
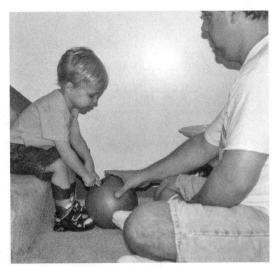

10.26   *10.27a*   *10.27b*

Follow your therapist's directions and have your child reach up or out to either side only if it is recommended.

Sitting and Reaching Down

1. Help your child sit on a bench placed in front of a couch or on the first step of your stairs (if of the right height).
2. Kneel or sit in front of her.
3. Help her to sit with her knees apart and her feet flat on the floor.
4. Encourage her to lean forward and then come back up as you play with her.

The boy in photos 10.27a and 10.27b likes to hear the air stream out of the ball. He will change between sitting straight and leaning far forward as his dad moves the ball.

Many other activities may be used for this activity. For instance, you may hold Mr. Potato Head and place the pieces for it next to your child's feet. Now she can lean forward and down to get a piece and come up to put it in its place. Similarly, she may play with a puzzle.

Wheelchair Posture and Balance Exercises

Older children who use a wheelchair continue to benefit from exercises in bench sitting. As they improve their sitting posture and balance, they become able to shift their sitting position and use their hands better for table work. Maneuvering and steering the chair or moving in and out of the wheelchair with as little assistance as possible are important functional goals for them.

For convenience and safety reasons, children who use wheelchairs may do the exercises while sitting in their chairs. Use them as recommended by your child's therapist.

1. Your child sits in her wheelchair with the wheels locked in place.
2. Sit in front of her and remove any chest support. Loosen, but don't open her seatbelt, move her slightly forward and wedge a tightly folded or rolled towel between her lower back and the backrest of the chair.
3. Encourage your child to sit tall without leaning against the backrest.
4. Prop a puzzle board on your child's lap, hold up a puzzle piece, have her reach for it and put it in its place. Have her reach forward and to the sides. Encourage

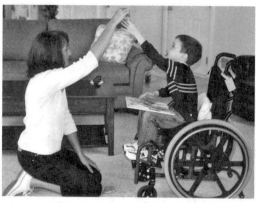

10.28

her to shift her weight in the direction she wants to reach before she stretches her arm out. Have her reach with either hand (photo 10.28).

5. Hold out a ball, have her lean forward and reach for the ball, and then toss it away.
6. Together with your therapist, look for suitable bench sitting exercises for your child and adapt them for wheelchair practice.

Note: Tighten the seatbelt and refasten any chest supports before you step away from your child even momentarily.

Moving in and out of Bench or Wheelchair Sitting

The first activities in this section train moving from sitting to the floor and from the floor into sitting. They are for small children who cannot yet stand independently or for older children who use a wheelchair. The second set of activities trains children who sit down from standing or get up to stand.

Before practice you may model the activity for your child using a large doll or stuffed toy. Make it interesting for her to watch and stress problem solving. "Teddy sits on the couch. He cries 'I want to get down!' Teddy impatiently wiggles around and falls down. 'Oh no, Teddy, that's not the way to get down! Place both hand to one side...." It will help your child to be familiar with the movement sequence before you practice it.

Sliding Off the Couch

1. Have your child sit and rest against the back of the couch.
2. Encourage her to turn, place both hands to one side (photo 10.29a), roll onto her tummy, and slide down feet first (photo 10.29b). Assist her as needed.
3. Have her pause as her feet touch the floor. Help her as needed to stand leaning against the couch (photo 10.29c) and then lower herself into the floor.
4. If the couch is too high for your child to slide off easily, make it lower by taking the cushions off. Later, after she can do it well, have her try to slide off with the cushions in place.

"This was easy," the girl in the photo tells us with her smile.

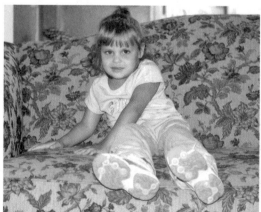

10.29a

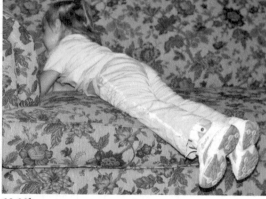

10.29b

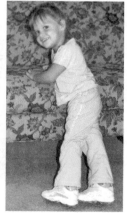

10.29c

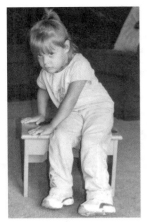

10.30a

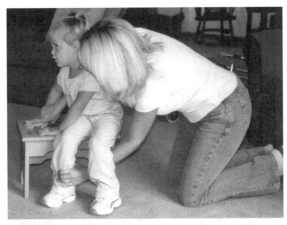

10.30b

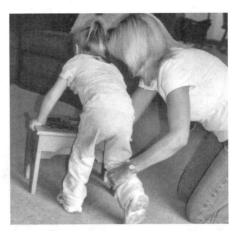

10.30c

Getting Down from a Bench

1. Your child sits on one side of the bench.
2. Have her turn to the free portion of the bench and place both hands there (photo 10.30a).
3. Assist with her hand and foot placement (photo 10.30b) and guard her with your hand at her chest as she swivels off the bench (photo 10.30c).

Moving Out of the Wheelchair

1. Start with your child sitting securely in the chair.
2. Lock the chair. Remove the footrests or swing them out of the way. Remove any chest support and loosen but do not open the seatbelt.
3. Ask your child to turn to the left and grasp the left armrest with her right hand.
4. Stand very close in front of her, open the seatbelt, help her turn her trunk, and slide down with her tummy toward the wheelchair.
5. Assist her to pause and stand as her feet touch the ground.
6. Next assist her into kneeling and then sitting on the floor.

After your child is familiar with the activity, help her less. Only when you are sure that your child will be safe, have her slide out off the wheelchair on her own as the boy shown in photos 10.31a-d is demonstrating.

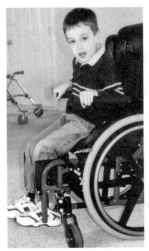

10.31a

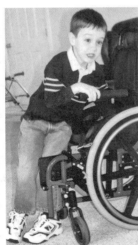

10.31b

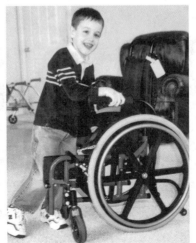

10.31c

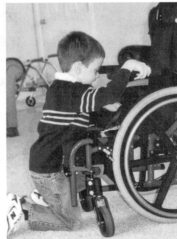

10.31d

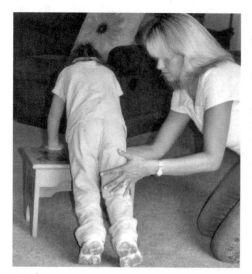

10.32a

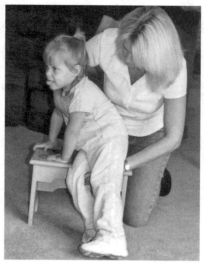

10.32b

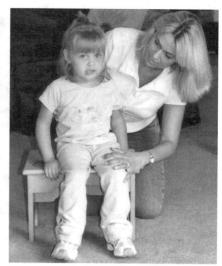

10.32c

From the Floor to Bench Sitting

1. Have your child crawl to the bench and place her hands on it.
2. Help her as she comes up and places her feet on the floor (photo 10.32a).
3. Help her move her hands (photo 10.32b) and swivel into sitting on the bench (10.32c).
4. As your child improves, reduce your support and only secure the bench for her until you feel she can safely do it all on her own.

From the Floor into the Wheelchair

1. Lock the wheelchair and remove or swing out the footrests.
2. From a bunny position on the floor assist your child into tall kneel.
3. Help her reach up and hold onto the armrests.
4. Help her place one foot forward, and push into standing.
5. If your child is tall enough, have her hold onto the edge of the backrest with one hand and an armrest with the other hand, and pull herself with your assistance into her chair.

After your child is familiar with the activity, help her less. When she is ready, have her do it on her own as demonstrated by the boy in photos 10.33a, b, and c.

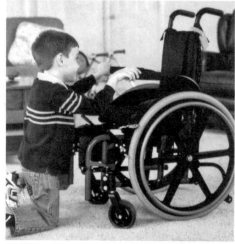

10.33a

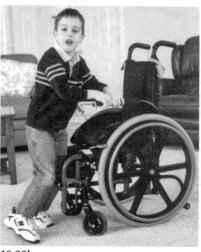

10.33b

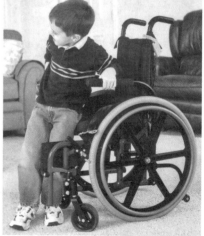

10.33c

Frequently Asked Questions

Q. *"When my daughter, Amy, sits propped up on her arms, her hands are fisted. The therapist wants me to open her hands each time I have her sit this way. I feel this is useless because she will fist them again a little while later. What do you think?"*

A. Follow the therapist's advice. Even though Amy keeps her hands open for only a brief period, each brief period will add up to helpful training. When she props up with hands fisted, she is using all her arm muscles instead of just the ones needed for the job. When her hands are open, her arms are more likely to work as they are supposed to.

Q. *"Amy has soft splints, which keep her thumbs out. Should she wear them when she sits with arms propped?"*

A. Yes, it will make it easier for her to keep her hands open and hold herself up without stiffening her arms. The longer Amy sits with hands open, the stronger and more coordinated her arms will become.

Q. *"Brittany always w-sits. Her therapist says it's bad for her. But Brittany will not listen to me if I tell her to sit differently. What do you recommend?"*

A. You are not alone with this problem. Other parents have faced it. Once w-sitting has become a habit, it is next to impossible to change it. Children are comfortable in the position and are able to play well when w-sitting. But there are several strategies you can try. Whenever Brittany sits for a long period of time—for instance, when watching TV or a video or during circle time in school—have her sit differently. Try having her sit with weights or tailor sit. If these positions do not agree with her, have her sit in a small chair. Whatever you decide on, be firm about it.

When she is playing on the floor, correct her position only when you are playing with her. In my opinion, constant reminders during free play do more harm than good. Brittany may feel that you are constantly picking at her and you do not want to do that nor have her feel this way. You may as well relax. Take comfort in the fact that no study has shown that some w-sitting is harmful.

Q. *"Miles does not like to sit with sandbags over his thighs. Soon after I place them on him he pushes them off. I stopped using them and instead I put my hands on his thighs when he sits. Don't you think that is just as effective?"*

A. Sure, if you have the time and do it a lot. The only drawback may be that you will not notice his progress as much. It is difficult to remember over time how much support you give. If you use weights you will know, for instance, that a month ago you used five pounds and now three pounds will do.

Q. *"How could I get Miles used to the weights?"*

A. Whenever you use them, be sure Miles is ready to sit and play. Also, make sure that he does not take them off when you walk away because he wants your attention. Therefore, see how he does when you sit in front of him and play with him. You may even try to cover them up. Maybe "out of sight, out of mind" will work. You may also use Miles's favorite video or DVD to distract him and as an incentive. Each time the weights are off, pause the video. When they are back on, the video plays again.

Q. *"Leif's physical therapist has him sit on a large ball and trains his sitting balance reactions this way. Leif thinks it's a lot of fun. Why are there no therapy ball exercises in this chapter?"*

A. To do therapy ball exercises requires skill and training. An inexperienced parent may endanger her child. If Leif's therapist wants to teach you one of these exercises, she will probably have good illustrated home instruction sheets available to give to you (Jaeger, 1997).

11

Getting Up and Crawling

Justin is two years old and cannot yet crawl on hands and knees. During his therapy session he practices crawling, but progress is very slow. It may take a year of training to reach the goal. "Will it be worth it?" his parents wonder. "Justin will be three years old by the time he crawls. No other child in his preschool class will be crawling. The other children will think he is a big baby and the preschool teacher will not want him to crawl. Yes, it is great if he learns to crawl, but will it be age appropriate?"

It is true that even in special education preschool programs, teachers may not like their three-year-old students to crawl. They like for them to sit and improve their cognitive skills to be ready for kindergarten. It is not uncommon for speech therapists to share this view.

The physical therapist seems to be the only person concerned about crawling. "Why should I listen to her?" Justin's mother may think. "The home program the therapist wants me to do is difficult and boring. Why bother?" "Because your child is never too old for crawling!" is the therapist's answer.

Being able to move independently on the floor is a very important skill that has life-long application. Getting up from the floor onto their hands and knees and crawling will help children become independent in many ways. The following story illustrates why.

Meet Jennifer

"Jen sits and plays all by herself," her mother tells the physical therapist. "Not for very long, though. Sometimes she plays several minutes; other times she topples over sooner.

She doesn't mind. When she is on the floor she loves to roll. She rolls everywhere—she even gets into things. Her twin sister, Jill, is walking and Jen likes to be up too. Yesterday Jill was playing at her toy kitchen and Jen wanted to do the same. I supported her in standing and she stood for a long time. They had fun playing together."

Jennifer is 20 months old. Like her twin sister, Jill, she was born prematurely. While her sister's gross motor development proceeded as expected, Jennifer's lagged behind. She was subsequently diagnosed with cerebral palsy. In other developmental areas, the sisters develop at a similar pace. Both are learning to talk and Jennifer is especially social.

During physical therapy, Jennifer practices the hand and knee position (therapists call it quadruped or four-point), sitting balance, sitting up, and kneeling with arm support. Supported by her therapist, Jennifer first holds quadruped briefly. A few months later, she maintains the position without help for half a minute and sometimes even a minute. In other areas, she does even better. With minimal support, she kneels at furniture, she stands leaning against a table, and, with the help of her therapist, she walks up to ten steps with a walker. Jennifer's parents are very happy about her progress.

Jennifer is now two years old. Her progress sounds very good indeed. It becomes less impressive, however, when you realize that she cannot pull herself up to kneel or stand. Nor can she sit up by herself or push herself onto her hands and knees. On her own, all she does is lie on the floor and roll. On her own, Jennifer is stuck on the floor.

Right now it seems not to matter much. Jennifer's loving parents are young, enthusiastic, full of energy, and always ready to help. If Jennifer wants to sit up, they position her. If she wants to stand, they support her in standing or place her in the gait trainer. Whatever the family does, Jennifer participates in fully. This is wonderful. But, someday…. Someday, Jennifer will be twelve years old and her parents will be ten years older. "Of course, by that time she will be able to get up from the floor," anyone would think. This is not necessarily true. Only if Jennifer and her parents work toward it will Jennifer learn it.

Children with cerebral palsy will not necessarily learn a new skill just because they get older. Time is not on their side. The opposite is actually true. Basic skills are harder to acquire, as the children get older. This is why early intervention is so important.

Sure, Jennifer's parents want her to become as independent as possible. With strong support from Jennifer's physical and occupational therapists it does not take long to convince them that they need to help Jennifer learn to get in and out of positions on her own. Mom sums it up well: "We are glad about the things Jen can do with our help. We will keep it up, but getting up on her own and crawling has to be the priority from now on."

Jennifer has already achieved a small part of her goal. Placed in position, she can hold herself up on her hands and knees. She does it the easiest way possible. In quadruped her hips and knees are bent so much that her bottom touches her heels. Therapists call it the "bunny" position. Indeed, children look like little bunnies ready to hop away.

For many children with cerebral palsy, this is their starting point for getting up from the floor. From the bunny position they can come up into short kneel, swivel into sitting, move to a true quadruped position and crawl, or pull up to tall kneel and to stand. The bunny position is the key to all this. No wonder her therapist had started to practice it early on.

Jennifer cannot get into the bunny position by herself. For now the therapist has to help her. As Jennifer lies on her tummy, the therapist lifts Jennifer's hips off the floor and helps her pull one leg and then the other up underneath her. Then she helps her push her chest off the floor and put weight on her arms. This is not easy. Jennifer's legs resist being bent and her arms are too weak to push up. Will she ever be able to do this by herself?

Hard work needs a big motivator. Jennifer is resting on her tummy. The therapist moves a large box filled with colorful balls close to her. "Jen, come up. Let's play at the box." The therapist helps her pull her legs up. "Come up and look!" she coaxes. Jennifer lifts her head and struggles to push up with her arms and lift her chest off the floor as the therapist helps her. Such a big effort has to be rewarded. The therapist quickly assists her to kneel at the box. Jennifer loves to look at the balls, touch them, and move them around. After a little playtime, the therapist puts her back onto her tummy. "This is a good situation. Let's take advantage of it," is her reasoning. Back on the floor, Jennifer knows what she wants. After the therapist has moved her legs up, she is ready to lift her head and push with her arms. Kneeling at the box, she has fun playing with the balls. Again and again, the therapist practices the same sequence.

Jennifer likes the activity and is working hard. Soon she needs less help with her arms and her therapist notices less resistance when she bends Jennifer's legs. Is Jennifer trying to pull them up? After seven repetitions, Jennifer is tired. It has been a good practice session—a good beginning. The next therapy session will be a little easier for Jennifer, and her parents can practice helping her come up.

From now on, coming to hands and knees is part of Jennifer's routine. Each time she wants to sit or stand, she is first helped to come onto hands and knees. The help is gentle—giving her time to do as much as possible on her own.

Several weeks later, no one remembers for sure when, Jennifer pushed up to quadruped for the first time on her own. At first, she did it only occasionally. Each time it became easier. With help from her therapist, Jennifer started to play in the bunny position. Supporting herself with one arm while playing with the other was another big challenge. She frequently tumbled to the side. Luckily, Jennifer did not mind. She continued to get into the bunny position. She would reach high to pull the magazine she wanted off the couch or even try kneeling at furniture. Now spills were potentially more serious. "I constantly worry that she will hurt herself," her mother sighed. "I have to watch her all the time." Then she mused: "First we worried that Jen was not doing enough on her own—now she is doing too much."

Indeed, Jennifer was daring. Pulling to kneeling or trying to heel sit was more than she could handle at the time. She did not have the balance, the trunk strength, or the shoulder, arm, and hip coordination. Instead of pulling up and endangering herself, it was time for Jennifer to not only come up onto hands and knees, but to learn to crawl.

When crawling on hands and knees, children constantly bear weight through their arms and shoulders, legs, and hip. They move arms and legs alternately one at a time. Their trunk is not resting on the floor, and all trunk muscles are working hard. Their balance is challenged with each crawling move. Crawling would give Jennifer the training she needed to become more coordinated and stronger, and to improve her balance. It would get her ready for other challenges.

Jennifer had her own opinions about crawling, however. She never had liked to move forward on her tummy. She had no urge to move forward on hands and knees.

To get somewhere, she rolled. Even if something was close by, she would go down on her tummy and roll instead of trying to crawl to it.

Not surprisingly, it took hard work, persistence, and a lot of patience for Jennifer to start crawling. She was three years old when she crawled across her play area for the first time. It took even more time for her to get good at it.

Was it worth all the effort? The answer is a resounding "yes." Jennifer has progressed so much. She gets up from her tummy onto hands and knees independently and crawls. She gained the ability to reciprocally move her arms and legs. She can sit up without help, pull up to kneel independently and pull to stand. She is learning to crawl up the stairs and pull to stand with more ease by placing one foot forward (half-kneel) as she gets up.

At the same time, her walking with a walker also improved. The arm strength and coordination gained by crawling help Jennifer be safe and steer the walker with ease. Now that her legs are stronger and more coordinated, stepping forward has become more fluent. Best of all, she is almost independent with her walker. With supervision and some help stabilizing the walker for her: she crawls to the walker, pulls to stand, turns around, walks where she wants to go, and lowers herself safely to the floor again. Jennifer's walker skills, however, did not improve automatically just because she learned to get up and crawl. They needed to be trained as well. Yet, success with her floor skills helped her accomplish the walker skills. Functional indoor and outdoor walking with a walker has become a realistic goal, which Jennifer may reach in the near future.

Up onto Hands and Knees

The story of Jennifer is not an unusual one for a child with cerebral palsy. While some children crawl with ease by the time they are two years old, others need as much help and training as Jennifer did.

The following are examples of how to work with children so they come up onto their hands and knees, hold the position, and learn to play or move in quadruped. Do the activities first with the help of your child's physical therapist and follow her specific instructions.

Getting Up Onto Hands and Knees

This activity shows you how to assist your child to get up from the floor onto hands and knees. Do it slowly and encourage your child to do as much as possible by himself. It will take time for your child to learn this. For most children, it is easier to hold a position on hands and knees than to push into it. Consequently, you can expect that your child will be able to hold the hands and knee position independently before he can push into it on his own.

1. Your child lies on his tummy and you kneel beside or behind him.
2. Slide one hand under his right hip and nudge his bottom up.
3. With your other hand, push his right leg up so his knee and hip are bent (photo 11.1a).
4. Push the left leg up the same way.
5. Brace his knees and hips between your legs while you help him to lift his chest off the floor, straighten the elbows, and place his hands (photo 11.1b).

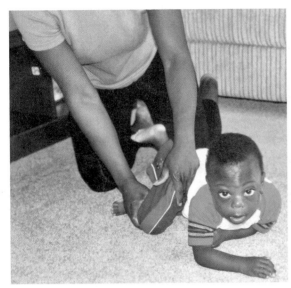

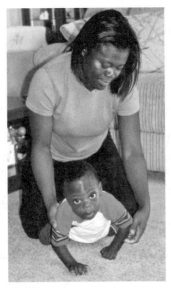

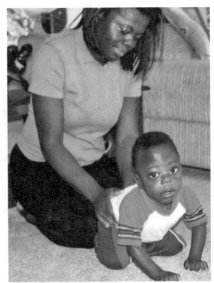

11.1a *11.1b* *11.1c*

6. Now push his knees a little closer together, adjust the feet so the toes point toward each other, shift his weight backwards (his bottom will be over his heels), and see if he can maintain the position with support to his hips (photo 11.1c).

Variation. After your child is used to the routine, try to reduce your support. After you nudge the right hip up a little, see if he will pull up the leg on his own. Do the same on the other side. Next, lift his chest some and see if your child will push himself into a bunny position.

Easy Hands and Knees (Bunny Position) with Hip Support

1. Help your child lift up off the floor onto his hands and knees as described above. See to it that his legs are bent as much as possible at the hip and knee. Most likely his bottom will touch his heels.
2. Keeping one hand under his chest, place an interesting-to-watch toy in front of your child (but out of his reach)
3. Remove your support to his chest, firmly hold his hips with both hands from the sides, and encourage him to stay propped up on his arms as long as possible.

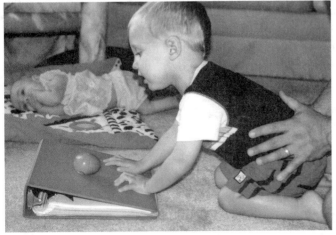

11.2

Variation A. If your child does not have sufficient arm strength or control to hold the position, place a wedge (a notebook binder may substitute for a wedge) in front of him and have him prop his arms up on the wedge (photo 11.2). Now less weight will be resting on his arms. Let something roll down the wedge. It will be interesting to watch and makes the activity fun for your child.

Variation B. If recommended by your child's therapist, have him wear soft arm splints while practicing this.

Note: When your child is on hands and knees, his toes should point backwards or inward towards each other.

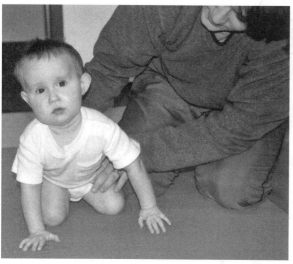

11.3

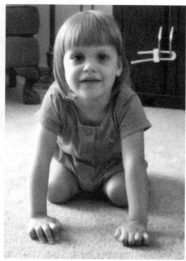

11.4

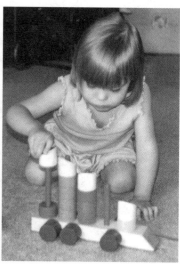

11.5

Quiet Rocking on Hands and Knees
1. As described before, help your child lift up off the floor onto his hands and knees.
2. Support his hips and gently rock him side to side (photo 11.3).
3. Next, rock him gently forwards and backwards. Be careful not to move your child more than a couple of inches forward until he has gained the needed arm strength and coordination.

Holding the Bunny Position Independently
1. As described before, help your child lift up off the floor onto his hands and knees.
2. After you are sure that his legs are bent as much as possible and his arms are placed well (as shown in photo 11.4), see if your child can hold the position without your help. Show him a picture book or whatever interests him and encourage him to stay up as long as possible.

Variation. After your child holds the bunny position well on his own, encourage him to bring his bottom up somewhat and shift more weight onto his arms. This brings him closer to a true hands and knees position as needed for crawling.

Playing on Hands and Knees
1. After your child is up on hands and knees, place an easy-to-play-with toy, like a roly-poly chicken or a pop-up toy, in front of him.
2. From in front of your child, encourage him to lift his right arm and tap the chicken. Be ready to support his left arm if needed.
3. Do the same with the other arm.
4. Do many repetitions.
5. If he does well, encourage him to play on his own with any toy of his liking (photo 11.5).

Crawling, One Move at a Time
1. After your child is on hands and knees, place something interesting a foot out of reach. Place the item on a stool if your child immediately tries to roll or crawl on his belly to it. Tell him: "Let's crawl to it."

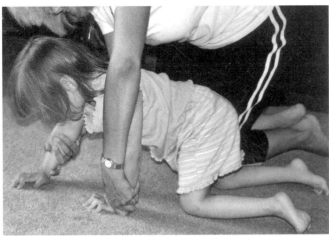
11.6a

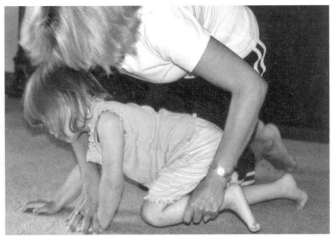
11.6b

2. Help your child move his right arm forward a couple inches and then move his left leg a small step (photos 11.6a and 11.6b).
3. Next move his left arm and help him step with his right leg. If your child wants to slide both arms forward at once, hold one hand in place with your hand while you encourage the other to move. Stabilize one knee if he wants to move both legs forward together.
4. Repeat the crawling pattern until your child reaches the toy. Repeat the sequence as often as your child likes to.

Note: Watch your child. As soon as you notice that he moves an arm or leg on his own, stop assisting him with that arm or leg.

Crawling

When children first start to crawl, they will do so in various ways. They may move first their arms, then the legs, either one at a time or together. They may move the arm and leg of one side of their body and then of the other side. Or they may start out crawling reciprocally—moving the right arm and the left leg and then the left arm and the right leg. Whatever they do, their movements will be choppy and unsteady. They need time to sort it out.

After your child has been crawling a few days or weeks, you will notice that he will use a more consistent pattern. If this means that he always scoots forward with both legs at a time, talk to his physical therapist for advice. You want your child to

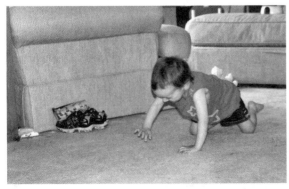
11.7

alternately move one leg at a time and develop a coordinated reciprocal crawling pattern. This will prepare him for alternately stepping forward—as we do when we walk.

As soon as your child crawls well on his own, encourage him to crawl everywhere. You want to build up his stamina and endurance. You want him to crawl for longer and longer distances. Remove clutter from the floor and give him an open space for practice. Soon your child will be able to crawl from room to room (photo 11.7). He will enjoy exploring his environment better than he ever could by rolling or crawling on his tummy.

Of course, he will get into things you don't want him to. So be sure to "childproof" your house by locking up cleaning supplies, using baby gates and socket covers, etc.

As he becomes more coordinated, obstacles will no longer deter him, but will become a welcome challenge. He will crawl around some and over others. After some practice, he may even crawl over your stretched-out legs. On a nice day you may take your child outside and encourage him to crawl in grass. Most likely he will be hesitant at first, but crawling on an uneven surface like a lawn will be good exercise. You may also have your child practice crawling up and down an incline. A sloping lawn or a ramp will provide this challenge.

Next, encourage your child to crawl fast. For fun, have a sibling race with him after a ball. If the sibling is older, tell him to let your child with cerebral palsy win sometimes. The more speed the better. The ability to move his arms and legs fast will be a very useful skill when he starts walking. Fast walking requires less balance. Beginning walkers have poor balance and may compensate for it by taking quick steps. Frequently they start walking this way and only later learn to walk slowly.

Eventually, your child might be ready to crawl up the stairs (photo 11.8). This is not easy and is dangerous when children try it alone. If your child is interested in crawling up the stairs, have him practice when you are with him. Guard him well as he goes up. When he wants to come down, do not have him crawl face first, but let him slide down on his tummy feet first (photo 11.9). He may object, but "feet first" is a safety measure all children need to learn.

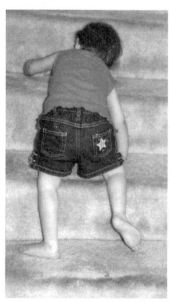 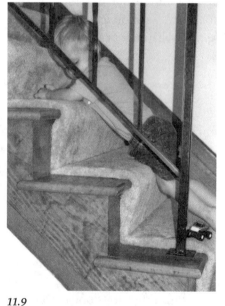

It may be boring and time consuming to watch your child going up and coming down stairs. You may be tempted to stop him. Don't! For your child, this is an adventure and it's great exercise. At this point, crawling up and down stairs gives him more of a workout than he may get at the playground or even during his physical therapy session.

There are no crawling exercises in this book because as soon as your child is able to crawl reciprocally on hands and knees he will find the "exercises" just right for him in his environment. All you have to do is allow him to take off, monitor his safety, and enjoy his antics.

11.8   *11.9*

Rising Up and Moving Down

Not all children start to crawl after they succeed in coming to hands and knees. Instead, some children pull to kneel, as Jennifer did, rise up to sit on their heels, or swivel into sitting on the floor. They learn what therapists call **"transitional" movements.** This simply means that they move from one position to another. So far they have mastered two transitions. They can turn from their back onto their tummies—they roll—and they can get up from stomach-lying onto their hands and knees.

The arm strength and coordination gained by pushing into quadruped now helps them to master the transition into or out of sitting, and pulling to a kneel. More hip and trunk strength and coordination will help them to make the transition into tall kneeling. Additional leg strength will allow for a transition to standing.

For you, moving from one position to another is easy. Yet, for small children, especially for children with cerebral palsy, sitting up is a major hurdle. They master it first by pushing up onto hands and knees, and from there they transition into sitting. Lowering themselves from sitting to stomach-lying on the floor is just as difficult for them. Indeed, what they master first—sitting up or going down—depends on a child's preference. A child, who likes to sit and play, will work hard to sit up by himself. A child who would rather move about will more likely figure out how to get down when he is placed in a sitting position.

The next activities show you how to help your child to sit up and move out of sitting. Use them as directed by your child's therapist and follow any specific directions given.

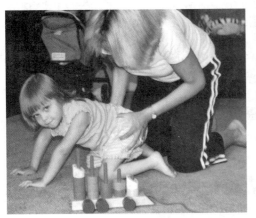 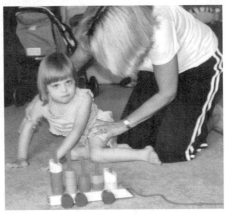 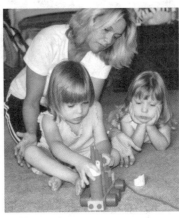

11.10a *11.10b* *11.10c*

Sitting Up

1. After your child has pushed up onto his hands and knees, place a toy to his left side.
2. Support his hips well and lower his bottom down to the right side (photo 11.10a). He will be in a side-leaning position with most of his weight on his right arm (photo 11.10b).
3. Encourage your child to bring himself forward and over toward the toy (photo 11.10c). Continue to support his hips as he struggles to sit up.
4. Repeat this activity with him sitting up over his left side.
5. As your child improves, reduce your support.

Encourage your child to sit with his legs out in front or have him tailor sit like the girl in the photo.

Moving Out of Sitting

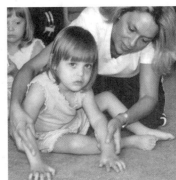

1. Your child sits on the floor.
2. Put a toy out of his reach to his right side.
3. Now have your child turn his trunk and place both of his arms to the side on the floor (photo 11.11).
4. Help him as much as needed to lift his bottom, come up onto his hands and knees, or lower himself to the floor.

11.11

Pulling to Kneeling

1. Your child is on hands and knees in front of a sturdy toy box filled with interesting things. For stability you may kneel behind him and brace his legs and hips between your legs.
2. Encourage him to shift his weight over one arm, reach up with the other, hold onto the rim of the box, and pull to kneeling (photo 11.12). If he struggles, place your hand over his hand so it will not slip off the rim. Try not to support his chest. You want him to do as much as possible on his own.
3. Once he kneels at the box, encourage him to keep holding onto the rim with one hand while playing with the other hand.

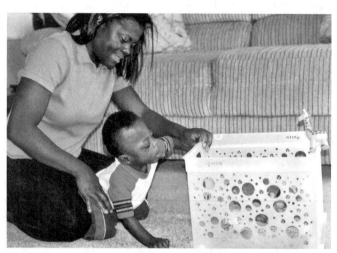

11.12

For a child who can hold a position on hands and knees without help or who crawls independently, pulling to kneeling at a sturdy box may be easy.

Guard or support him as needed from the side but do not sit or kneel behind him. Initially, your child may lose his balance backwards. If you are behind him, he will feel safe, lean against you, and will not learn to prevent a backwards fall.

Moving into Heel Sitting

After your child can kneel with arm support, he may be ready to heel sit.

1. From hands and knees, encourage your child to shift his weight backwards into a bunny position.

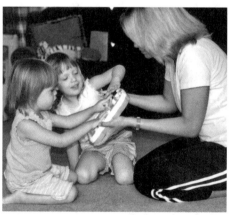 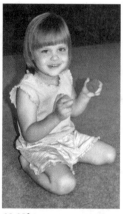

11.13a   11.13b

2. Kneel in front of him holding a busy box or another sturdy, interesting toy he likes.
3. Encourage your child to sit back on his heels, come up, and play. In the beginning your child will lean onto the toy as he plays. Later, discourage him from doing so by tilting the toy or holding it vertically (photo 11.13a). This way he will heel sit and play with less support.
4. Later have him hold a small toy and see if he can balance and heel sit all by himself (photo 11.13b).

Doing It All

Most children learn to crawl, sit up, pull to kneel, and improve their balance in sitting and kneeling all at the same time. As they get better with these skills and gain more independence, parents may notice changes in their children's behavior. A quiet, passive, at times moody child may become an active, outgoing little fellow who is interested in his environment.

Many children with cerebral palsy enjoy crawling and playing on the floor by two years of age. Both you and your child will be happy that he is now independently moving about, playing on his own, and no longer has to be constantly helped and carried from room to room.

Savor it! Your child will benefit from lots of crawling. His arms, legs, shoulders, hips, and trunk will get stronger and more coordinated as he learns to crawl faster, to kneel straighter, and to transition from one position to another with ease. It will help him with standing and walking—but not if his leg muscles are allowed to shorten.

The two-year-olds who crawl and kneel look so cute. Parents relax and think of them as "cured." If your child is one of those cute children be glad about it, but do not forget his daily leg stretches. And do not forget to work on pulling to stand, standing with arm support, and stepping. As the "Road to Independence" in Chapter 4 describes, it is best to work on these skills at the same time your child practices sitting and crawling.

Typically developing children sit, then crawl, stand, and finally walk. They master the skills in sequence. So you expect the same from your child with cerebral palsy. "Why then the rush into standing? My child just started to crawl," you wonder. It is best to practice standing and stepping concurrently with kneeling and crawling. It assures that his knee and ankle joints remain flexible. It teaches your child to weight bear over his feet as well as over his knees. It saves time and assures that no opportunities for standing will be missed.

As you already know, your child needs more time and practice to learn motor skills. He may be three years old or older before he sits, kneels, and crawls well. To start standing and stepping practice at age three is late. By that time your child may not like to stand but rather be independently crawling. Between one and two years is a good time to start standing practice. At that age, children like to stand. It is a good time to lay the foundation for this important skill. The next chapter helps you to do this.

As soon as your child crawls on his own—you no longer have to practice it with him—start to emphasize standing. Practice it daily as directed by your physical therapist.

Frequently Asked Questions

Q. *"When Josh crawls, he does not move his legs alternately but scoots forward with both at the same time. What can I do?"*
A. It will be best if you ask Josh's physical therapist. He knows Josh and can give you specific advice. A general recommendation is to have Josh practice crawling in places where scooting is difficult and where you have some control over the situation. You can spread a large blanket or quilt on the floor and see if this discourages Josh from scooting. During the warm season, have daily crawling practice on your lawn. Scooting is difficult there and Josh may let you help him to reciprocally crawl to an interesting target. Most likely, Josh is not able to scoot up an incline. With your help have him move up one leg at a time. If you have stairs in your house make it part of his routine that he crawls up with your help. The more Josh uses his legs reciprocally, the easier it will become, and the more likely he will crawl this way on his own.

Q. *"When Audrey crawls, she fists her hands. Should I be worried about that?"*
A. Most likely fisting will be a temporary occurrence. As Audrey crawls more and crawling becomes easier for her, you will notice that her hands will fist less tightly and

eventually open. At the same time there are things you can do that will help Audrey. Practice open-hand weight bearing with Audrey. Ask for activities that practice it if Audrey's therapist has not yet given you any.

Does Audrey have soft hand splints? If she does, make sure she wears them. The splints help her to open her hands and she will be more likely to crawl without fisting.

Q. *"Melissa likes to hold things in her hands when she crawls. Is this bad for her?"*
A. No, it shows that Melissa has progressed with her crawling skills and is now able to carry her favorite things along with her.

Q. *"Naseri sits up without coming first onto his hands and knees. Is this wrong?"*
A. No, while most children sit up by first coming onto their hands and knees, some push into sitting from stomach-lying. Children who sit up this way have flexible hip joints and show good coordination of their hip, trunk, shoulder, and arm muscles.

Q. *"Braden loves rolling around. He finally learned to crawl but he still rolls most of the time. What should we do?"*
A. Most likely rolling is still easier for Braden than crawling. Do not scold him for rolling. Observe when Braden is most likely to crawl and make the most of these situations. For instance, will he crawl out of narrow spaces when you play with him? Is he more likely to crawl in the kitchen than in the living room, or is it the other way around? Have him spend more time in the room he prefers to crawl in. Hallways are great places for crawling. Have Braden play there and encourage him to move about by placing his favorite toys at different ends of the hall. Instead of verbally reminding or praising him for crawling, you want him to take ownership of his new skill and use it because he wants to.

12

Leg Exercises and Standing with Arm Support

The previous chapters gave you many activities and exercises to strengthen your child's arm and shoulder and trunk muscles. This is because children primarily use these muscles when they learn early functional skills. They use them to push off the floor into sitting, kneeling, and onto hands and knees.

"Shouldn't I also exercise my child's feet and legs as early as possible?" you may wonder. Yes, of course. Most likely you have already been doing so. When you played with your child in back-lying and did a *Spine Curl Up* or *Happy Baby Plays with Feet* you started to exercise your child's legs. Whenever you diapered and dressed your child, you touched and moved her legs, and this too stimulated muscle activity.

Sensation is important. Sensation stimulates movement. You know your arms are sensitive to touch, but your legs are too. The palms of your hands have a special keen sense of touch and so do the soles of your feet. When you walk barefoot on gravel you quickly experience how sensitive your feet are.

Your child's legs and feet are sensitive and when you touch them you stimulate muscle work. If your child plays with her feet or if she touches the floor with them, this too will encourage foot and leg muscle activity.

The first advice to parents who want to stimulate their child's leg movements is very simple. It requires no work or time, but rather saves both. It even saves money. This is the advice: don't cover your child's legs unless it is necessary, and **never cover her feet unless it is absolutely essential.** Sleepers, which hide your child's feet, are all right for sleep but not for daytime when your child is active. You want your child to see her feet and toes and move them freely. For the same reason, don't cover her feet with socks. Little socks look cute, but don't have your child wear them except on special occasions or when she is wearing shoes. Socks do to feet what mittens do to hands—they greatly reduce the sensation you receive. Mittens interfere with everything you want to do with your hands and get in the way of your sense of touch. You don't have your child wear mittens all day long. You know it would hinder the use of her hands. Likewise, try not to use socks indoors. Her foot muscles will develop better without them.

"But my child will get cold feet!" you object. Yes, without socks her feet may be cold. But as long as her thighs are warm, you do not have to worry. If you worry nevertheless, have her wear two pairs of long pants during extra cold days.

"But my child needs shoes!" you decide. Shoes hinder and restrict your child's feet even more than socks do. Shoes are meant to protect your feet when you are walking. **As long as your child does not pull to stand or walk, shoes have no function. They are just an adornment and a hindrance to your child's gross motor development.** In shoes, children cannot stretch or curl up their toes freely. These movements strengthen the muscles of the feet and stimulate leg movements. All these spontaneous movements are good. They help the muscles get stronger and more coordinated.

"But won't shoes help my child to stand and walk?" you counter. I may smartly answer that shoes possess no magic and will not make your child stand and walk. It takes balance, sufficient leg strength, and coordination to walk. This is correct, but it is also true that shoes and good ankle braces make a difference when your child stands and walks.

Children with delayed motor skills usually have very weak ankle and foot muscles. Children with cerebral palsy often have not only weak but also spastic calf or foot muscles. Both the weakness and the spasticity make it difficult to place the feet and hold the ankle joint in the best position for standing and walking.

The feet and the ankle joints are your base when you stand. This base affects your standing posture. Changes of your base and your standing posture may cause balance problems and even a fall. For instance, if your calf muscles are very weak, your ankle joint may bend far forward, causing your knees and hips also to bend, possibly causing you to fall down forward. Tight, spastic calf muscles may cause the ankle joint to bend backwards, which causes the knee to bow backwards or the heel to be pulled off the floor so that the children stand on toes. Correct, good fitting ankle braces and shoes will lessen these ankle problems and provide your child with a better base of support. For some children, the braces are not only helpful, but essential for standing and walking. The last chapter will provide more details about this.

Even though shoes and braces help children with cerebral palsy to stand and walk, they hinder them when they are crawling or playing on the floor. This poses a problem because most children with developmental delays or cerebral palsy will engage in all these activities for several years. Like Jennifer, they may learn to crawl on the floor and to walk with the walker at the same time and their parents want to give them good opportunities for both. Taking shoes and braces on and off several times a day may prove to be the only solution. This is extra work for parents, daycare workers, or preschool teachers, yet if you want to foster motor development, it is essential. As your child becomes more capable, you can teach her to help with this chore.

Stimulating Leg Movements

The following are more ways to stimulate leg movements:

Start leg range of motion exercises with your baby as early as possible. They are easy to do and most children like them. The exercises are done at three different speeds. At the slow speed, you move the legs through their full range of motion and mildly stretch the muscles. At the faster speeds, you move the legs as far as they go with ease, which will be less than full range. The exercise is meant to stimulate active movements and keep the hips, legs, feet, and toes limber. Practice them first with the help of the physical therapist and do the faster movements only if your therapist recommends them.

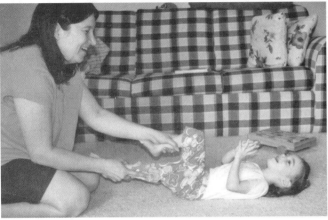

12.1

Kicking the Legs Slow and Fast

Do this exercise after each diaper change.

1. Your child lies on her back.
2. While you hold her left leg down, bend her right knee and bring it up toward her tummy (photo 12.1). Pause.
3. Move her right leg down and hold it down while you move her left knee to her tummy. Pause.
4. Repeat two times.
5. Repeat this several times at a faster pace without pausing, creating a fluid kicking pattern.

Ankle Rolls and Wiggle Each Toe

Do the exercises as described in Chapter 5, *Flexible Muscles and Joints*.

Happy Baby Plays with Feet and Independent Play in Back-lying

You also want your child to lift her legs up on her own—together or one leg at a time. Hand-to-foot play will do this. It strengthens the muscles that bend the hip, stretches the muscles that straighten the hip, and improves coordination. This, in turn, will make it easier for your child to roll over, crawl, and later walk.

Have your child do the activities as described in Chapter 7, *Happy Baby in Back-lying*.

Intermittent Pressure through the Leg

This exercise is for children who do not yet stand with support. It lets them experience pressure through their ankle, knee, and hip joints—similarly to the way it would happen if they were standing. Do the activity only if recommended by your child's therapist.

1. Your child lies on her back with her legs straight.
2. Cup your right hand around her right heel and place your other hand lightly over her right knee (photo 12.2).
3. Give gentle, intermittent pressure into her heel. Direct the pressure through her ankle and knee joints into her hip joint. With your left hand, make sure that the knee does not bend.
4. Give intermittent pressure through the left leg similarly.

12.2

Leg Exercises

So far you have helped your child to move her legs. Now you want her to do as much as possible on her own. Some of your child's muscles may be especially weak and benefit from extra training. The muscles that bend the hip joint are often weak in children with cerebral palsy. They are strengthened when the children lie on their back and raise their legs against the pull of gravity. The next four activities encourage children to lift their legs high in playful ways. Small children as well as older children who still need to improve their hip strength and coordination may enjoy them.

If you therapist recommends the exercises for your child, use them according to any specific instructions given.

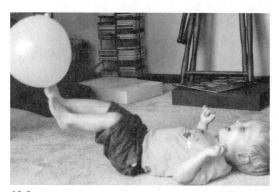

12.3

Kicking a Balloon

1. Hang a balloon or light ball from the ceiling with a string and have your child lie under it on her back.
2. Have her kick the balloon as hard as she can. Encourage her to make it fly up as high up as possible (photo 12.3).

Start with the balloon hanging low and close to her feet. You want her to be successful, have fun, and enjoy doing it again. As your child gets better after a week or two, challenge her by hanging the balloon higher.

Kicking with One Leg

1. Hang a balloon or light ball from the ceiling, as before.
2. This time, hold one of your child's legs down on the floor and ask your child to kick with the other (photo 12.4).
3. Repeat this exercise holding the opposite leg down

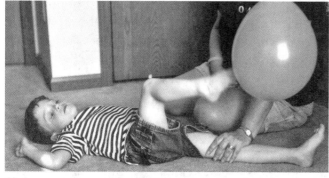

12.4

Note: Kicking with one leg requires more leg muscle control than kicking with both. Momentum from whole body movements cannot assist the effort. With one leg pinned to the floor, the other leg has to do all the work and its hamstrings will be stretched. Hang the balloon in just the right spot for easy kicking. You want your child to have fun and do this very effective exercise with "gusto" again and again.

Lift the Ball

1. Your child lies on her back.
2. Hold a lightweight ball over your child's legs.
3. Have her grab the ball with her feet, bring it up toward her chest, take it with her hands, and then toss the ball away. If needed, help her by placing the ball between her feet and holding it there, and then bring her legs up high enough so she can reach the ball with her hands (photo 12.5).
4. Later, reduce your support and have her do as much as possible on her own.

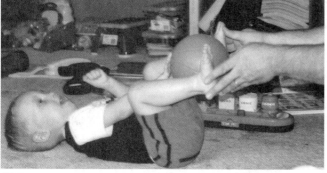

12.5

Foot through Ring

1. Your child lies on her back.
2. Give your child a ring (as used for a ring toss game or diving) and challenge her to bring her left foot up and put her foot through the ring (photo 12.6). If she cannot do it, help her hold the ring up and lift her leg by pushing her thigh up. Have her practice again and again until she can bring her foot through the ring with as little help to her leg as possible.
3. Repeat and have her put her right foot through the ring.

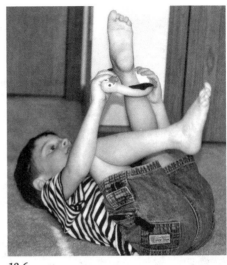

12.6

Scooting Backwards

For older children who are able to sit on their own, the following activities may be used to train specific leg muscles. Use them as directed by your child's physical therapist.

Have her practice the scooting activities in a large recreation room, a hallway, or in your driveway. If a sibling joins the activity it will be more fun.

1. Your child sits on a scooter board,
2. Have her hold onto the board with both hands, and move backwards by pushing off with one foot at a time.

Scooting backwards trains the hip flexors and the quadriceps muscles. (The quadriceps is the big muscle on top of the thigh.)

Note: Scooting backwards is easier for most children then scooting forward, which is listed next. But there is the danger of a backwards fall when your child scoots backwards. You want to be mindful of this and be sure your child can handle the activity before she practices in the driveway.

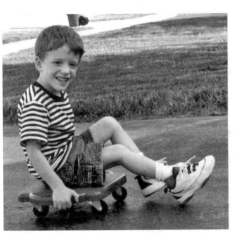

12.7

Practice the activity first on a level surface. An incline will make it harder to control the scooter. Only when your child is ready for the challenge, have her try it on a sloping driveway (as demonstrated by the boy in photo 12.7).

Scooting Forward

1. Your child sits on a scooter board.
2. This time, encourage your child to move forward by stretching one leg out, pushing down with the heel while stretching the other leg forward, and so on.

Scooting forward trains the hip flexors, the quadriceps, and the hamstring muscles. (The hamstring is the big muscle at the back of your thigh.)

Kicking in Sitting

1. Your child sits on a bench with feet flat on the floor and braces herself with her arms on the bench.
2. Dangle a balloon on a string above her foot.

3. Ask her to slide her right foot forward, and tell her to kick the balloon. Have her kick the balloon as often as she likes (photo 12.8a).
4. Repeat, having her kick with the left foot.

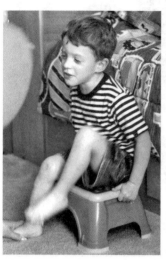

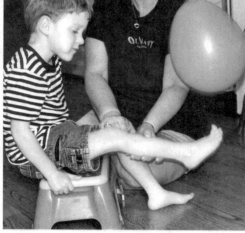

12.8a   12.8b

Kicking the balloon will train your child's quadriceps muscle.

Variation. If your child has difficulty kicking with one leg at a time, change the exercise as described here.

1. Tape the balloon string to the tabletop and have the balloon dangle down from the kitchen table.
2. Have your child sit on a bench facing the table with her stretched out right foot underneath the balloon.
3. You sit at the left side of your child and firmly hold down her left leg with her foot flat on the floor. Encourage your child to kick the balloon with her right foot. If needed, assist her in bringing her right foot up a few times and then let her try on her own (photo 12.8b).
4. Repeat and have your child kick with her left foot.

Supporting Your Child in Standing

As children develop, they pull to stand and are typically able to stand at furniture between 8 and 10 months of age. Most children with cerebral palsy are not able to do so until much later. Yet, it would be good for your child to experience standing at the same age. Standing stimulates leg muscle activity; it stretches and activates the muscles of the ankles and feet, and puts healthy pressure through the bones and joints. Weight bearing in standing causes calcium to be deposited in the child's leg bones, and, as a result, the bones become denser and stronger.

Children are born with soft bones, which contain little calcium. Throughout childhood, the calcium content of the bones increases. The children are depositing calcium into their "bone bank." Three years after growing stops, young adults have achieved peak bone mass in their "account" and can "draw" from it later in life.

Children, who never stand, deposit far less calcium in their bones. They are at risk of developing bones that break easily. Even short periods of standing are beneficial. Active standing, where the weight is shifted from one leg to the other, is better than standing still.

Often it is not easy to place and support your child in a good standing position. Having her stand with poor posture (with a forward leaning or backwards arching trunk, or standing on toes) will establish bad habits and reduces her chances of learning to stand independently later. You need to work with your child's therapist and follow her advice about ways to encourage good standing.

A child shows a good standing posture when both feet are well grounded, flat on the floor with toes pointing forward or slightly outwards. The hips and knees are straight and in alignment with the shoulders (photo 12.9). The child may lean slightly forward but *not* backwards.

The following are two examples of how to place and support your child in a good standing posture. Practice the activities first with the help of your child's therapist and follow any specific instructions she recommends.

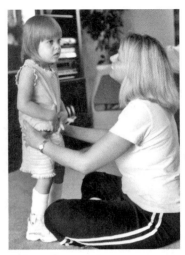

12.9

Standing with Support

1. Sit on a low stool or chair. Support your child as she stands sideways between your knees and lower legs (photo 12.10).
2. With your hands, make sure that her hips and knees are straight and her feet are planted firmly on the floor—a bit apart and with toes pointing forward or slightly outward.
3. When your child stands with good posture gradually support her less with your legs, so that most or all of her weight is upon her legs. Assist her at the knees if her legs start to buckle or turn in.

Variation A. If your child's legs buckle or turn in whenever they bear some weight, observe which leg is most likely to do so. Have your child stand with her weaker leg closest to you and support the knee of that leg firmly with both hands.

As soon as your child is able to stand for a longer period of time, do the activity in front of a table with some toys for her to play with.

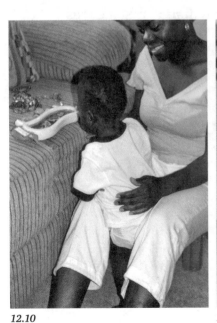

Variation B. If buckling of the knees is a persistent problem, your child's therapist may suggest that your child wear knee immobilizers while standing. Have her lie on her back while you put the immobilizers on.

As before, have your child stand between your legs in front of a low table. Your child may still slightly bend her knees in spite of the immobilizers. But it will be easier for you to help her stand with her hips and knees straight part of the time. Encourage your child to play with toys on the table and stand as long as she likes.

Variation C. If it is difficult for you to have your child stand sideways between your legs, try supporting your child facing away from you as shown in photo 12.11.

12.10   12.11

Standing with a Lean-To Board

If supporting your child in standing is especially challenging, a padded board for your child to lean against may help. (See the Appendix for instructions to make the board.)

Place the board slightly forward, slanted against your couch or another suitable piece of furniture.

Have your child stand and lean against the board while you support her from behind. Encourage your child to play in this position for several minutes.

The child in photo 12.12 does best if he is allowed to stand on Mom's legs.

Note: Support you child at all times when using the board.

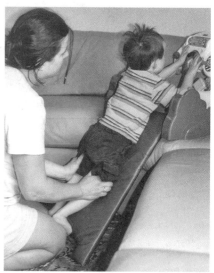

12.12

Supported Standing with Weight Shift

1. Sit on a low stool and support your child between your knees and lower legs as she stands facing you.
2. As she bears weight, make sure that her legs are in a good position—feet flat, a bit apart, and toes pointing forward or slightly outward (photo 12.13).

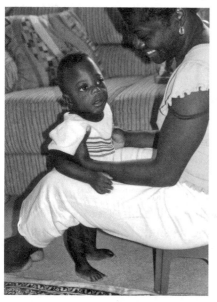

3. Now hold her with both hands around her chest and move her slightly to the right side so most of her weight is on her right leg. Pause.
4. Move her back to the middle and then to the left side. Pause.
5. Move her back to the middle and then a little forward. Pause.
6. Repeat 10 times, creating a rhythm. Play some music with it for fun.

Variation A. If your child tends to come up on toes, try the following: Take your shoes off and place your feet over your child's feet. The weight of your feet may be all it takes to keep her feet in place.

Variation B. Once your child is able to do the activity well, you may accent the weight shift by giving some downward pressure during each pause. This encourages her to bear all her weight first over the right and then over the left leg. If the downward pressure causes her knees to buckle, lighten up, or discontinue the pressure.

Note: Do not do the forward movement if it causes your child to bend her hips or come up on toes.

12.13

Leg Exercises with Weight Bearing

Leg exercises in standing will not only strengthen your child's leg muscles but also train the coordinated up and down movement pattern at the hip, knee, and ankle joints. As soon as you are comfortable supporting your child in standing, her physical therapist may recommend one of the following exercises.

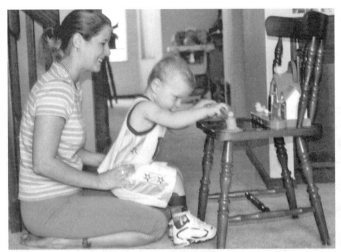

12.14a

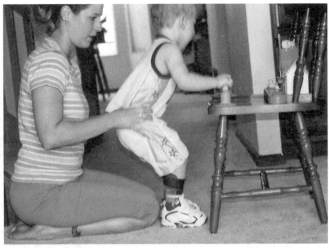

12.14b

Sit-Stand-Sit with Support from Behind

A bar suctioned to the surface your child stands at will make the exercise easier for a beginner. Holding on and pulling with her arms, she can assist her legs as they

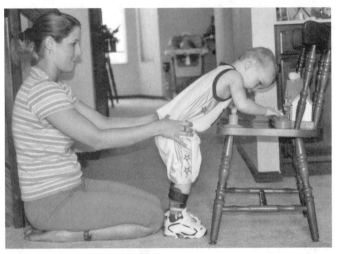

12.14c

push up. (A suction bar may be purchased in a hardware store or ordered from a pediatric equipment catalogue. See the Appendix.)

1. Place an interesting toy on a table or sturdy chair of a good height (about waist high to your child). Suction the bar at the edge closest to your child.
2. Kneel in front of it and have your child sit on your leg (photo 12.14a). Direct your child's attention to the toy. Have her lean forward, grab the bar (photo 12.14b), and stand up (12.14c). Provide as much hip support as needed for safety.
3. Later, encourage her to lean forward and push her bottom backwards. Help her as needed to bend her hips, knees, and ankles and sit down again.

Sit-Stand-Sit with Your Child Facing You

1. Your child sits on the first step of the stairs or on a stool. (Or, as in the illustration, a shoebox can make a low seat.)
2. Sit or kneel facing your child. With your right hand, hold both of your child's hands. Your left hand stabilizes her right hip and thigh from the side (photo 12.15a).
3. Pull your child forward and up into standing (photo 12.15b) and then have her sit down again. Pause.
4. Repeat many times or as long as your child enjoys the exercise. Prompt her by saying: "up"; "down."

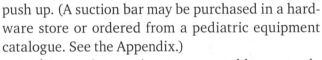

12.15a   12.15b

Variation. If your child pushes mostly with one leg (stronger), do the following: Adjust the position of the other leg (weaker). Make sure that the hip, knee, and foot are aligned and the foot points forward. Place your free hand on the hip and thigh of the weaker leg for extra assistance as your child moves up and down.

Initially, your child's attempts to stand up and sit down will be very jerky. The more you practice the exercise, the smoother the movement will become.

To lure your child to come up, put a small toy, a ring, or beanbag on your head.

Note: *Your child should not push backwards when standing up.* Do not use the exercise if pushing backwards cannot be prevented.

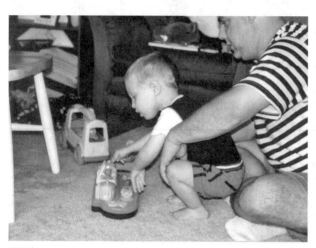
12.16a

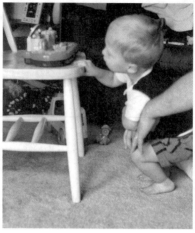
12.16b

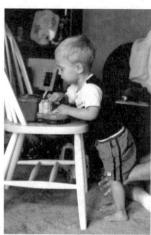
12.16c

Squat-Stand-Squat

During this leg exercise, the child also moves up and down with your help. It is well suited for children with increased muscle tone. Use the exercise only as directed by your therapist, follow her instructions, and be sure to practice with the therapist's help before you attempt it at home.

1. Place a kitchen chair close to the play area. Put your child's favorite toy on the floor nearby.
2. Help your child to squat down in front of the toy with feet flat. Assist your child by holding her knees apart and out. Encourage your child to relax, lean forward, and play a few minutes (photo 12.16a).
3. Briefly support your child with only one hand while pulling the chair in front of her. Put the toy on the chair.
4. Ask or help your child to reach up with one or both hands (photo 12.16b) and to push into standing. Place your open hand between her knees if she tries to push her knees together in standing (photo 12.16c).
5. After about a minute of standing, move the toy back to the floor and help her to squat down again.
6. Repeat as often as your child likes to play.

Your Child Stands Holding on with Both Hands

Your child stands well when you support her and she likes it. "Is there a way she could stand by herself?" you wonder. If your child already crawls and sits independently, the physical therapist will soon show you how to help her pull to stand at furniture and play while standing. On the other hand, children who cannot crawl and sit will not be ready for this. As explained in Chapter 13, children first gain balance in sitting and kneeling before they are able to acquire it while standing. ***Children are not able to stand without arm support before they can sit independently.***

However, even children who cannot sit independently may learn to sit as well as stand holding onto a bar. They may learn the following sequence: from sitting holding onto a bar they pull to stand, hold onto the bar as they stand, and then they lower themselves back down into sitting—still holding on. This may be a very difficult activity for your child. It may take time, and much patience and training, for your child to be able to do this. Yet, your child's proud and happy smile as she stands all by herself will be worth the effort. Unfortunately, because she needs to hold on all the time, she will not be able to play while standing. Nevertheless, standing with arm support is a very useful skill, especially for children with more severe types of cerebral palsy.

The earlier children learn to stand this way, the better. Pulling to stand and standing holding onto a bar will enable them to assist with dressing and toileting. It will make it possible for them to move (transfer) from one chair to another (or to their bed, etc.) on their own or with minimal help. They will become more independent as they incorporate "transfer skills," as therapists call them, into their daily routine. When they are grown, and lifting them becomes difficult or impossible, these transfer skills will be very important.

The following describes, step-by-step, how to teach your child to stand up, stand, and sit down while she holds onto a bar. It is important that you practice this first with the help of your child's therapist. Only after your child is participating well and the therapist directs you, may you do these activities at home.

Equipment. You will need a stool or bench for your child to sit on and a bar to hold onto.

The seat has to be of the right height so your child's feet rest comfortably on the floor. For a small child, a twelve-pack of canned soft drinks may make a perfect seat. For an older child, a stepstool or an upside-down storage crate may be just right. Place the seat in front of a bar she can reach and grasp onto, and then use to pull herself up into a standing position.

A bar such as a towel bar or bathtub safety bar attached securely to the wall will work well. Right under a window would be a good place to attach it. This way your child may look out as she stands. The bar should not be too thick but just right for your child's hand to grasp. Christopher's parents attached a bar for Christopher to stand at in their family room and there he practices standing. Another option is a bar with suction cups that can be suctioned to a smooth surface. This kind of bar may be ordered from a therapy equipment catalog (see the Appendix).

If you do not have a bar for your child to use, look for something stable and easy to grasp. Your child may hold onto the top of a playpen, the slats of a crib, the rungs of a ladder-backed chair, or the edge of a weighted down trashcan or clothes hamper.

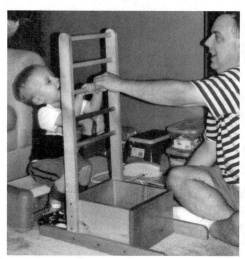

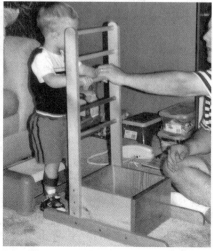

12.17a   12.17b

Put magazines, old phone books, or a stack of newspapers into a new trashcan or hamper so it will not tip over.

If you would like to have a special piece of equipment for your child to pull up to, you may build a ladder box as seen in photos 12.17a and 12.17b (see the Appendix for dimensions) or purchase a walking ladder (also called Peto ladder). The ladder is available through pediatric therapy equipment catalogs.

Standing while Holding On with Both Hands

1. Help your child to sit on a stool with her feet shoulder-width apart, flat on the floor, and toes pointing forward.
2. Have her lean forward, reach up, and hold onto the bar with both hands. Be at her side and place one hand over hers to ensure that they don't slip off the bar (photo 12.17a). With your other hand be ready to help your child lift up off her seat. (Work with your therapist to find the best way to assist your child.)
3. Tell your child: "lean forward, push up, and stand." As she stands, praise her, and have her stand by herself while still securing her grasp around the bar (photo 12.17b).
4. When she is ready, help her to sit down slowly, while still holding onto the bar.

Some points to remember when you practice this activity with your child:

- Do not have your child pull to stand with her arms only. Instead have her lean forward, putting weight over her feet, and push to stand with her legs, and not just pull up with arm strength alone.
- Have your child hold onto the bar (or top edge of a trashcan, playpen, etc.) with both hands at all times. The goal of the exercise is that your child learns to stand up, remain standing for a period of time, and sit down all by herself and do it safely.
- If you use a weighted trashcan or hamper for your child to pull up at, she may want to lean with her trunk against it. Do not allow this, as it may tempt her to take her hands off. This is very unsafe. A child who does not yet sit or kneel independently is in constant danger of falling if she does not hold on well.
- When your child no longer wants to stand holding on, have her sit down and end the practice session.

After your child is able to pull to stand, as well as stand and sit down with your help, you want her to do it by herself. Here are some goals you can set to pace your child's progress.

1st Goal: Holding on with both hands, your child stands up and sits down without help.

When your child stands up or sits down, try to reduce your assistance except for safety reasons. Continue to secure your child's hands with yours. Guard her well from the side (photos 12.18a and 12.18b). The emphasis is not on standing for a long time but on practicing five or more repetitions of up/down.

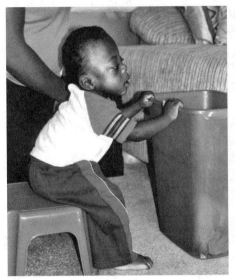 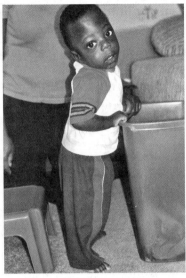

The more your child practices, the easier it will become and the more likely she will no longer need your boost coming up or your help holding on going down. Be prepared for it to take several weeks of daily practice to achieve the goal. It will test your imagination to motivate your child to come up again and again. "Come up and give Mommy a big kiss" may work for a while, but after Mom has gotten kisses on both cheeks, and Teddy one on his snout, your child might tire of this game. If nothing else seems to work, pieces of favorite foods may do the trick.

12.18a *12.18b*

2nd Goal: Holding on with both hands, your child stands safely for 30 seconds.

Now you can make standing fun and motivate your child to stand longer. Praise her for standing straight and tall, have her sing a song with you, or play music while she stands. You may even encourage her to wiggle side-to-side with the music. It is fun and gets her to shift her weight from one leg to the other— something she needs to learn. Starting out, make sure her hands don't slip off as she "dances." Guard you child well from the side while she is standing.

You may be surprised how long 30 seconds are. It may take several days or weeks of daily practice to reach this goal. It may get tiring to entertain your child as she practices standing. After a while, you both will be ready to work on the last goal.

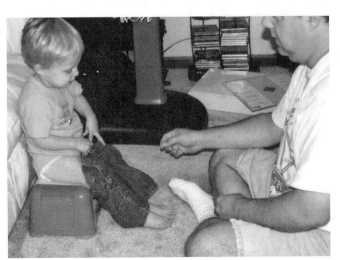

3rd Goal: Holding on with both hands, your child stands during daily tasks.

Think of times it may help you if your child stands. For instance, when she gets dressed in the morning, you can have her sit while you put her pants over her feet, then she can pull to stand, and you pull her pants up while she stands. If your child uses a wheelchair, her therapist may give you a transfer task to work on.

Once you have decided on your child's daily standing tasks, make them as convenient as possible for you. Set up a "standing station" in the bedroom, bathroom, family room, or wherever your child will be standing (as illustrated in photos 12.19a and

12.19a

12.19b). You have succeeded when supervised standing is no longer an exercise but a useful task that helps you with your child's daily care.

In summary: Standing, holding on with both hands, benefits bones, joints, and muscles; it enables children to be more independent, and it boosts their self-esteem. Children with more severe types of cerebral palsy will benefit from it all their lives. Other children may improve their balance, first in sitting and kneeling, and then also in standing. For these children, standing while holding on with both arms bridges the gap between the time they are ready for standing and when they have the balance to do so without holding on.

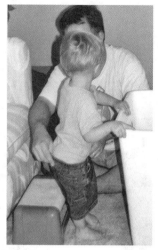

12.19b

Helpful Bars

Frequently children with cerebral palsy show limited improvement with their standing balance. They learn to stand well with one-hand support but have difficulty standing with no support. If they have good arm and hand strength they like to hold onto sturdy bars. It makes them feel secure and allows them to do things they otherwise would not be able to. For young children, bars allow for efficient training of standing and stepping skills. For older children, bars may make it possible for them to be independent with personal hygiene.

A Banister along the Wall

Banisters are longer and sturdier than bars. Their brackets space them away from the wall. For young children, they make a good station for practice of pulling to stand, standing balance, and stepping (photo 12.20).

For older children, a banister in the hallway provides security as they put on a coat, grab their book bag, and head out of the door with their walking aid.

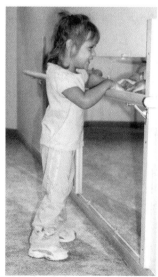

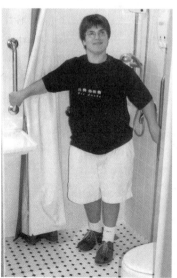

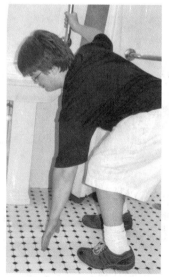

Grab Bars in the Bathroom

Grab bars in the bathroom provide personal freedom and privacy to older children. In photos 12.21a and 12.21b a teenager shows off his bathroom. "It is so convenient. Wherever I am I have a bar to hold onto. I leave my forearm crutches by the door when I step in

12.20   *12.21a*   *12.21b*

here," he tells us. "If I drop something, I hold on and pick it up. It's easy, much easier than when I have only a crutch to hold onto."

Frequently Asked Questions

Q. *"In back-lying, our son Julian kicks his legs really well. We tell him: "Kick, kick, kick" and he kicks up a storm. Shouldn't this help him to walk?"*

A. Yes and no. Yes, because moving his legs on his own is good and will help Julian. No, because the kicking pattern is different from a walking pattern. The patterns may look alike but they are different. Kicking is an alternating up and down movement pattern. Walking is about stepping out and moving forward. In order for Julian to walk, he has to learn to move his legs in other ways too.

Q. *"My daughter Madison stands very well when I hold her around her knees and pull them backwards, so her legs are straight. Madison's body leans a little forward, but she keeps her hips and back very straight. Why don't you recommend this exercise to parents?"*

A. I do not recommend this type of standing because it encourages the child to use only the muscles at the back of her body to stand up. When Madison stands as you describe, she uses the muscles at the back of her thighs, the muscles at the back of the hip, the back muscles, and the shoulder extensor muscles. For good standing and balancing in standing, Madison has to use the muscles at the front of her body and at the sides of her hips as well. Holding herself up just with her back muscles establishes a habit that will hinder her when she wants to move, bend down, reach, or take a step.

Q. *"My son's therapist is able to help Tom pull himself up to stand really well. But at home he cannot do it. I help him so much but he still does not pull to stand the right way. What should I do?"*

A. Don't feel inadequate about this. Be patient. Your therapist has been helping children for years—it's no wonder it is easier for her. Have your spouse, a relative, or a friend assist you. Ask your helper to accompany you to Tom's therapy session. This way they can observe the therapist and both of you can practice with the therapist's help.

Q. *"You recommend that children do not wear braces during floor play. I have three students in my preschool class who wear AFOs. I like to follow your advice but find it is far too time consuming for me to take their braces off and on. What do you suggest?"*

A. You are right that it takes time to take shoes and braces off and back on. There is no good solution. You may delegate the task to your aide or volunteer. If you do this you have to make sure, however, that your helper knows how to put the braces on. You may ask the physical therapist to teach her how to do this correctly.

13

Balance

What is so special about our ability to balance? We are in balance when we sit or stand and our center of gravity is over our base of support. A plastic doll, if placed just right, may be balanced so that it can stand. Yet, there is a difference between the doll and us. We can actively shift our weight and move our center of gravity, while an inanimate object cannot.

Let's see what this means. A strong breeze swishes by—the doll falls down—but we don't. We are constantly adjusting our posture and keeping our balance when conditions in the environment change. No healthy person is blown over by wind.

Now, bend the doll at the waist and see what happens—it falls over. We do the same and we don't lose our balance. Why? Before we bend forward our muscles are busily working. They shift our body backward, counterbalancing our forward movement. We do this without conscious effort. Our brain (our central nervous system) directs the muscles to work preceding all voluntary movements.

Regardless of how our balance is challenged—by the environment or by our own movements—our muscles are ready and working to keep us upright. They do so with as little effort as possible and without voluntary command. A special organ in our middle ear, small receptors in our joints and skin, and our vision perceive information about our body's position, and send it to the brain, where it is processed and then sent to the muscles for action. This all happens very fast, within a split second. How steadily we balance depends on how smoothly this process works, and how well each part functions.

If the sensory input or information we get is poor, we don't balance as well as we otherwise could. Try standing on one leg, first with your eyes open and then with your eyes closed, counting how many seconds you are able to balance. I am sure you do better with your eyes open. This demonstrates how important vision is for balance and explains why a person with good vision has better balance than a blind person or someone with poor vision. Also, when we look at quiet surroundings, it is easier to balance than when we look at moving objects or people.

If a person has poor muscle coordination and muscle weakness, he will not balance as well as a strong person with good coordination. This explains why a frail elderly person is more likely to lose his balance and fall than a healthy athlete is.

Balance in Children with Cerebral Palsy

Children with cerebral palsy have poor balance. How much their balance is affected varies from child to child. There are several possible reasons for balance problems:

1. The deficiency may be caused by the fact that children with cerebral palsy are unable to produce the fine-tuned muscle work needed for balancing.
2. Difficulties may be due to interfering abnormal reflexes.
3. The brain may not properly process information about the body's position in space and/or send out the information needed by the muscles to react to this information.

Problems may also be due to a combination of all these factors.

Some children with cerebral palsy seem unable to perceive when they are in danger of falling. Others appear to be acutely aware of their body's position, understand that their muscles are not doing their job, and grow anxious and frightened during an activity that requires balance skills. These children may overreact to a perceived balance loss and thereby further endanger themselves.

Balance skills emerge like gross motor skills in head to toe fashion. As children develop, they first become able to balance their head and trunk for sitting; the head, trunk, and thighs for kneeling; and finally the whole body for standing. Children with cerebral palsy develop balance skills in the same order.

How well children balance depends on their experience and how well their nervous system and muscles function. A person with extensive training of standing on one foot, like a ballerina or a gymnast, has better balance than a person without this training. This makes sense, although scientists have previously disputed this. Today it is proven that experience makes a difference and is even required for the development of balance skills. This is true for typically developing children and for children with cerebral palsy. Recent research showed improved standing balance in children with cerebral palsy following standing balance training sessions (Shumway-Cook, 2003 and 2005).

Knowing how difficult it is for children with cerebral palsy to develop balance skills, we want to provide them with the best opportunities for practice and lots of training.

Balance Training

During balance training your child works mostly on his own, without your physical support. It is best not to touch him unless the exercise directions call for it. Your job is to guard your child from the side and provide safe surroundings. If your child loses his balance, you want to be close enough to prevent a fall and assure that he does not get hurt. ***Do not stand behind your child during balance work.*** It will give him a false sense of security, which may actually increase his risk of falling when he tries the same activity by himself at a later time. If a situation requires you to be behind your child, make sure that he attends to something in front of him.

Safety is most important. You want to make sure that your child does not fall and get hurt. When your child tries something new and difficult, stay very close to him. Be ready to quickly and calmly support him when necessary.

Be a good observer. Your child's posture and his movements will tell you when he is insecure and may need immediate help or when he is safe. The more you work with your child, the better you will become in detecting these signs. You will be able to judge his progress and know when he gained the balance so you can step aside and have him safely try an activity on his own.

Be patient. Balance activities are more difficult than they appear to be. Doing many repetitions of basic tasks will build confidence. If you notice that an exercise is difficult and frustrating for your child, make it simpler or do not use it until you have had a chance to talk to your child's therapist about it.

Be aware that it is easier to balance in a quiet environment where nothing moves and no noise distracts. Calm, relaxed concentration helps your child to accomplish a new balance task. After he has gained confidence, have him do the activity when other people are present. As he learns to cope with distractions, he firms up his new skill.

Balance Training in Sitting

The chapter *Sitting Pretty* showed you how to help your child sit independently. With the biggest hurdle accomplished—your child can sit on his own—you may look for ways to further improve his sitting posture and balance. You want your child to be able to sit and lean far down, reach up with both hands, reach far forward, far to the side, and turn his trunk without falling. Training his sitting posture and balance will allow him to do more for himself at home and in school.

Use the exercises as directed by your physical therapist. The first two will "wake up" the trunk muscles and get them ready for more work. Boys especially like these exercises.

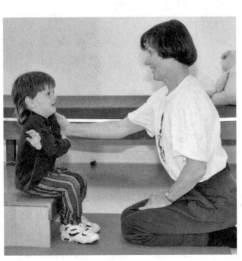

13.1

Stay Up

1. Your child sits with his feet flat on the floor and his knees not touching.
2. Tell him to fold his arms, sit straight, and be strong.
3. Say to him: "I am a mean guy who wants to push you down—don't let me." Give very mild pushes with your open hand to your child's trunk—to the sides, forward, backwards, and diagonally (photo 13.1). Start with slow, light pushes, increase the pressure, and then give quick taps. Adjust the pressure to your child's ability to withstand it. You want to challenge your child without causing a loss of balance.
4. Do three sets of ten pushes.

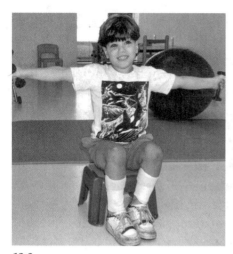

13.2

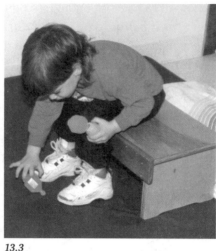

13.3

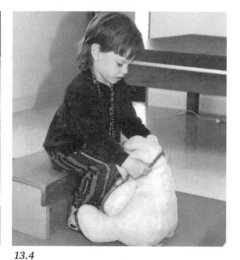

13.4

I Lift Weights

1. Your child sits with his feet flat on the floor and his knees not touching.
2. Put a half-pound weight in each of his hands. If you do not have little barbells, you may make a hand weight. Take an old sock, put some beans or rice in it, and close it by making a knot at the open end.
3. With your guidance, have him train like the "big guys." Count with him as he does 5 arm (biceps) curls, lifts his arms 5 times out to the sides and 5 times up (photo 13.2). Does he want to do more? Let him exercise as much as he likes.

Let's Make a Snake

Does your child sit without putting weight on his feet—do his feet seem to float over the floor? The following activities make him bear weight on his feet as he stretches and reaches far down. Try to find additional activities that provide the same practice.

1. Your child sits with his feet flat on the floor and knees not touching.
2. Place pop beads on the floor and have your child reach for them one by one as he builds a long snake (photo 13.3). If needed, help him push the beads together.

Let's Dress Up Teddy

1. Your child sits with feet flat on the floor and his knees not touching.
2. Place your child's favorite toy or stuffed animal by his feet.
3. Encourage your child to lean down and dress it up with necklaces, a hat, etc. (photo 13.4).

Press the Squeaker

1. Your child sits with feet flat on the floor and his knees not touching.
2. Place a soft, squeaking dog toy under your child's foot.
3. Encourage him to press down and make it squeak (photo 13.5). If he cannot do it, tell him to lean forward and press down on his knee with his hands. Let him make as much noise as he likes, giving each foot a turn.

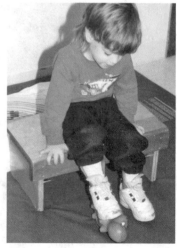

13.5

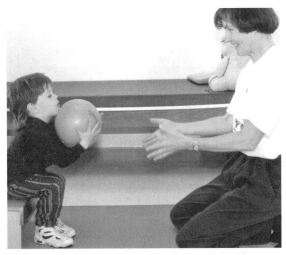

13.6

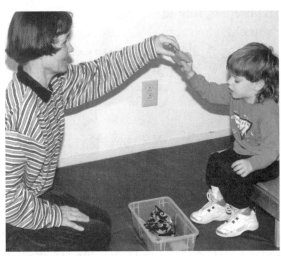

13.7

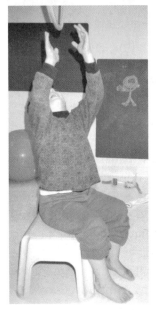

13.8

Playing with a Ball

Ball playing challenges your child's balance and is more difficult than you may think. Make it easy and fun. The more your child likes it, the more he will exercise.

1. Your child sits with his feet flat on the floor and his knees apart.
2. Choose a lightweight, medium size ball. Gently roll the ball to your child and let him roll it or pick it up and throw it back to you.
3. Next, throw the ball to him (photo 13.6): "Are you ready? Catch!" Start out by dropping the ball into his hands. "Good catch."

Beanbag Toss

For this game you need beanbags and a wide bucket, storage bin, dishpan, or similar container.

1. Your child sits with his feet flat on the floor and his knees not touching.
2. Place the bucket just in front of his feet.
3. Start by holding a beanbag within easy reach (photo 13.7). "Here, drop it in the bucket."
4. Next, hold it a little further away. But don't spoil the game by holding the beanbag too far away and frustrating him. Instead challenge him, keep holding the bag as he grasps it, and let him pull it out of your hand. Have your child reach with either hand. Make reaching high, to the side, and turning part of the game.

Throwing beanbags is fun for children of any age, especially if the target is well placed—neither too far nor too close. Emphasize the throw. Keep score to keep the game going. This will make your child eager to play often.

If your child only wants to use one hand, it may work if you let him hold something with this preferred hand. Get his favorite action figure: "Hold Jeff. He wants to watch you throw." Be ready to make adjustments for the not-preferred hand. The target, as well as the beanbags you hold out for him, will need to be closer.

Reaching with Both Hands

Challenge your child to reach up with both hands. This requires more weight shift and is harder than you may think. Use the activity only as directed by your child's therapist and follow any specific instructions given.

1. Your child sits with his feet flat on the floor and his knees not touching.
2. Something large and light like a hoop or a beach ball provides a good incentive for your child to reach with both hands. Place it on the floor for him to pick up, have him stretch for it as you hold it up (photo 13.8), or just let him play with it. Using both hands will challenge his balance.

Balance Training in Kneeling

Soon after or at the same time as children with cerebral palsy start to sit independently, they may also learn to kneel. The children first kneel with their hips bent. In this position, their hips rest over their legs—they short kneel or heel sit. The balance requirements for short kneeling are very similar to those needed when sitting on a bench; the trunk muscles do most of the work.

From short kneel the children learn to pull up to tall kneel. Now the hips are straight and only the knees and lower legs rest on the floor. Balancing in tall kneel requires the coordinated effort of the trunk, hip, and thigh muscles. This is something they have not done so far. They need much practice as they slowly acquire the skill with arm support; some children progress to tall kneeling without arm support.

Tall kneeling is a useful skill for children with cerebral palsy. It allows them to reach further and higher. As they move up and down, into and out of tall kneeling, their hip and thigh muscles become stronger and more coordinated. All gains made in tall kneel will be useful when your child practices standing and walking.

The subsequent activities will help your child to improve his balance in kneeling with the hips straight. The first two will encourage your child to rise to tall kneel. Use them as directed by your child's therapist and follow any specific instructions given.

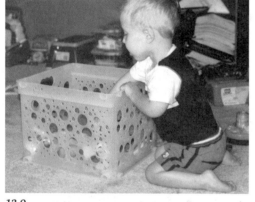

Play at the Toy Box

1. Get a sturdy toy box. An old-fashioned wooden box is good, but a plastic crate will do if you place something heavy like a telephone book on the bottom so it will not easily tip over.
2. Put some interesting things in the box and encourage your child to crawl over to it, pull up, and play. Be at his side to make sure he does not lose his balance to the side or backwards.
3. As you become assured that your child is safe, have him play independently at the box (photo 13.9).

13.9

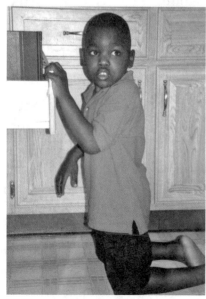

Play at a Drawer

1. Select a drawer in the kitchen or bedroom that he can easily reach up to.
2. Place things your child likes to play with in the drawer. Stand a tall box or book on end in the drawer, and tape it to the side corner of the drawer to keep it open.
3. Encourage your child to pull up on the drawer and look inside it (photo 13.10). Be with your child initially to make sure he is safe. When he is ready to play by himself, give him plenty of opportunities.

Your child may choose to play in heel sitting and not try to pull to tall kneel. "Should I help my child pull to tall kneel?" you may wonder. In this situation it is best not to worry. Let your child play however he likes. Children are curious. It is only a matter of time before your child will struggle up to look at what's hidden at the bottom of the box or drawer. Such an initiative, precious and memorable, is what you and your child have been preparing for.

13.10

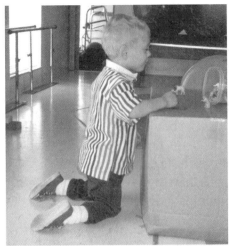

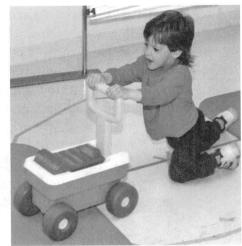

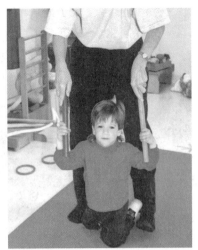

13.11   13.12   13.13

Play in Tall Kneel

As soon as your child is able to tall kneel, provide ample opportunity for him to practice. As he gains experience in the new position, his balance will improve. You will notice that it becomes easier and more enjoyable for him to play in the position.

- A couch or a coffee table may provide a good place for your child to play while tall kneeling.
- As your child improves, a large upside down cardboard box will make a good play table (photo 13.11).

Knee Walking Pushing a Toy Cart

When your child can crawl and play in tall kneeling, he is ready for this activity (photo 13.12).

Help your child to hold onto the cart (or other suitable walking toy) and stabilize it for him. This way he can get started slowly.

When your child knee walks pushing a cart, his hips are bent and the leg movements are similar to crawling, except the trunk is higher and only the legs propel him forward. Most likely your child will enjoy cruising around this way.

Knee Walking with Sticks

When your child walks in tall kneel, his trunk and hip muscles move in much the same way they do when stepping and walking in standing. The next activity encourages walking on knees with hips straight. Use it as directed by your child's therapist and follow any specific instructions given.

1. Get two sticks—a broomstick cut in half will do.
2. Have your child tall kneel. Stand behind him, holding the sticks at shoulder level on either side so he can grasp one with each hand.
3. Now, with both of you holding onto the sticks, go for a walk—your child on his knees in front and you right behind stabilizing the sticks and helping with weight shifting before each step (photo 13.13). If your child hangs backwards, try the same activity with you in front facing your child.

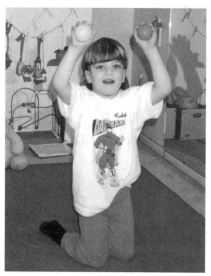

13.14

Tall Kneeling without Arm Support

Tall kneeling without arm support is very challenging for children with cerebral palsy. If your child's therapist recommends that you practice independent tall kneeling with your child, you may try this activity.

1. Your child heel sits in front of you.
2. Stretch your arms out and hold two small balls out of his reach. Encourage him: "Come up and get the bouncy balls" (photo 13.14). Wait for him as he struggles to come up. Lower the balls if needed. You want to reward his efforts even if he does not succeed.
3. After your child has tossed the balls, have him try to come up again.
4. Repeat as often as your child remains interested.

Some children are not interested in balls. "Reese likes to eat crackers," his mother reports. "Sometimes when he wants one of his favorite cheese crackers I tell him to come up for it and he does beautifully each time."

Standing Balance

In standing, your child has to control and balance his whole body—not just the head and trunk as in sitting, and the hip joint as in kneeling—but also the knee and ankle joints. When we stand, only the soles of our feet rest on the floor. This is our base of support. How large our support base is depends on the size of our feet, their position, and the distance between them. When children first try to balance in standing, they place their feet far apart, enlarging their base as much as possible. Still, they start out wobbly and frequently fall as they learn how to coordinate all parts of their body.

For children with cerebral palsy, standing brings unique challenges. They have to keep the hip and knee joints straight, the ankle joints in a neutral position (neither bent nor straightened), and maintain balance. If you have practiced the activity "Standing Holding On with Both Hands" with your child, you know he can stand straight and you may believe that standing with one or no hand support will be easy for your child to achieve. Unfortunately, this is not true. Standing straight is good for your child's joints and muscles but is not a good position to learn to balance in standing. As soon as the child lets go of the arm support, he is bound to fall backwards and get hurt.

Ten-month-old infants who stand at a table lean their trunks forward to prevent a backwards fall. Children with cerebral palsy try to do the same. Yet as they bend their hips to lean forward, their knees and ankles also want to bend, which would make them buckle underneath them. To stay up, the children stiffen their legs, which triggers the reflex pattern of scissoring. When scissoring, the hips bend slightly, the legs turn inward, push together, and the knees and the ankles stretch out. Children with cerebral palsy who show this pattern in back-lying are prone to rely on it in upright. Unfortunately, other children with cerebral palsy may also exhibit the pattern or a milder version of it (with less turning in of the legs) when standing.

When children use the scissoring pattern, they stand on their toes with their feet very close together and turned inwards. They are able to stand this way with support. Standing without support is another matter. Standing on their toes with their feet close together, their base of support is extremely small, making it impossible for them to balance.

Try it yourself and stand on your toes with knees touching. You can do it when you have something to hold onto; but without support you become very unsteady and feel as if you could lose your balance any moment. Try to walk this way up on your toes and with knees touching. It feels awkward but you can do it. Some children with cerebral palsy start out walking this way. It works for them as long as they are small. In the long run, however, this type of walking produces severe and lasting joint problems that may lead to an inability to walk by the time the child becomes a teenager or adult.

Standing and walking with a scissoring pattern is not a short cut that a child with cerebral palsy may use temporarily, but a dead end street. It does not lead to improvement and progress. Instead, it hinders the child from learning to stand without arm support and walk with a better gait (gait is a term frequently used by therapists and means walking pattern).

After your child is able to pull to kneel, you want him to learn to pull to stand, stand at the table without collapsing or scissoring, be able to play independently, and lower himself to the floor when he wants to. To accomplish this, your child needs special training.

How long it will take and how difficult the work will be, varies from child to child. It will take time and patience. The more you work with your child when he is initially learning to stand, the better he will learn how to stand—not compared to another child or to your effort, but to his potential.

You will have help with this task. Your child's physical therapist will work with your child and will guide the home program. Fortunately, today your child's doctor can also help you. He may prescribe braces that will support your child's ankle joints and set them in a neutral position. If your child's leg muscles are very hypertonic, the physician may prescribe medication or give injections directly into the muscles to reduce your child's muscle tone. All this helps, even though there can be negative side effects to consider. The medical treatment, its benefits, and its side effects are described in more detail in Chapter 17.

Whatever treatment you and your doctor decide upon, physical therapy and a home program will be the most important part of it. Ankle braces can help keep your child's feet flat on the floor instead of up on his toes. But wearing braces will not automatically make your child able to stand or walk. Physical therapy and your home program will train your child's coordination, weight shift, and balance. It will strengthen his muscles and keep his joints flexible. There is no brace, or pill, or injection that will do any of this.

Standing with Arm Support and Moving In and Out of Standing

If your child has high muscle tone and tends to stand on his toes, your therapist may recommend that you do the following exercises from Chapter 5 before practicing standing with him. They will loosen and stretch his ankle and foot muscles:

- *Ankle Rolls* and
- *Calf Muscle Stretch in Deep Squatting*

Do them as described in Chapter 5.

The standing activities below train your child to pull to stand, play while standing, and lower himself down to the floor. The best way to get into standing is by pulling to tall kneel, raising one knee forward and placing the foot on the floor (half-kneeling), and then pushing to stand. The same sequence in reverse order will help your child to lower himself from standing to the floor with control.

Pulling to stand via half kneel is difficult for most children with cerebral palsy. Tightness and weakness of the muscles that bend the hip may interfere with the forward movement of one knee while weight bearing on the other knee with the hip straight. Initially most children need much assistance with the task. As they gain strength and coordination, they gradually require less help. The training is very valuable for children with cerebral palsy. It teaches them to use one leg at a time and strengthens and stretches their hip and leg muscles. The goal is for the children to become independent with the task and integrate it into their daily life.

The next activities show how to assist your child to kneel on one leg and push to stand with the other leg, to place him in a good position for play in standing, and to get down from standing. Use them as directed by your child's therapist and follow any specific instructions he may give you.

If your child has ankle braces, have him wear them during the practice.

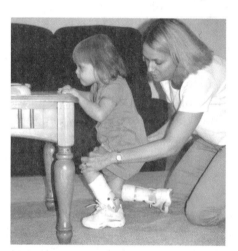

13.15

Half Kneel to Stand

1. Place something fun and easy to play with on the table.
2. Kneel behind your child and encourage him to reach up to the edge of the table.
3. After he has pulled to tall kneel, stabilize his right hip with your right hand from the side. Place your left hand at the side of his left thigh.
4. Help him shift his weight over his right knee, bring his left knee forward, and place his left foot on the floor.
5. Now place your left hand over his left knee and assist him to push into standing photo (13.15). Make sure his trunk leans forward as he stands up.
6. Have him practice standing up with the right leg the same way.

Variation. For more support, kneel very close to your child. Place your right hand in front of his right hip and stabilize it with your body from behind. Then proceed as before.

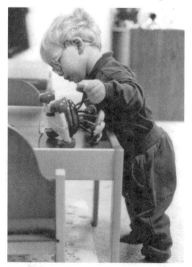

13.16

Standing with Play

1. As above, place something fun and easy to play with on a table.
2. Kneel behind your child and assist him to stand up via half kneel.
3. Help him to stand with feet flat on the floor and shoulder-width apart. His knees and feet should point forward or slightly outward.
4. As he stands well, move to his side and encourage him to play quietly at the table. Whenever your child turns his legs inward and rises up onto his toes, correct his position. Step behind him. Place your hands on top of his thighs and turn his legs slightly out. Ask or help him to stand tall and place his feet flat on the floor. If your child is about to lose his balance or becomes tired, help him to come down via half kneel.

A play table with an edge, as shown in photo 13.16, will allow the child to hold on for stability when needed.

The more quietly your child plays, the easier it will be for him to balance and to keep his feet flat on the floor. If it is difficult for you to place your child's heels on the floor after they rise up, your child's therapist will gladly show you how to do it.

Note: Remember not to be behind your child, as it tempts him to lean backwards against you. This only encourages him to remain dependent on you, instead of gaining independence.

Lowering to the Floor Via Half Kneel

1. Kneel behind your child. Place your right hand against the side of his right thigh and your left hand at the side of his left hip.
2. Ask or help him to shift his weight over his right foot, bend his left knee, and slide the foot backwards.
3. Assist his right leg as he slowly lowers himself into a half-kneel and then to kneeling. From tall kneel it will be easy to move into short kneeling, sitting, or to hands and knees.
4. Have your child practice lowering himself down with his left leg the same way.

Crouching Down to Sitting on the Floor

When ten-month-old children stand at furniture, they may lower themselves by crouching down and then dropping onto their bottoms to sit on the floor. Mastery of this movement sequence is also beneficial during a sudden backwards fall. If your therapist believes that your child will benefit from this skill, you may practice it as described below. A grab bar suctioned to the edge of the table will make the activity easier and safer for a beginner.

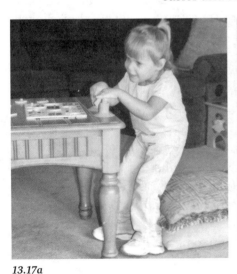

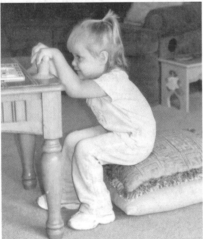

1. Place a couple of couch cushions on the floor behind your child as he stands.
2. When he wants to get down, ask him to hold onto the bar, lean forward, bend his knees (photo 13.17a), and sit down (photo 13.17b). Stand at his side and, if necessary, help him to bend his hips and knees.
3. When he is able to do this well, have him practice sitting down on just one cushion.
4. Finally, have him crouch low and sit down on the floor.

13.17a   *13.17b*

Crouching down is easier for the young children than going down via half kneel because they use both legs in the same way. It allows them to become independent earlier. As their legs become stronger and more coordinated, they then may learn to come down over half kneel.

Similarly, it is easier for many children with cerebral palsy to stand up from squatting or low sitting than from half kneeling. If moving into half kneel and then pulling to stand is challenging for your child, your therapist may advise you to practice the other ways of pulling to stand too. From squatting or low sit, your child pushes into standing with both legs. As he does so, he will gain strength, coordination, and balance control. All of this will help him to gain the ability to stand up independently in the future.

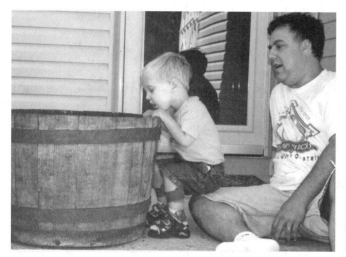

13.18a

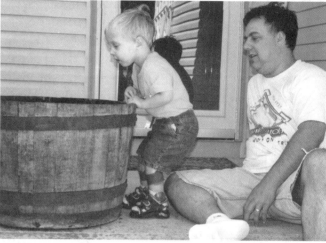

13.18b

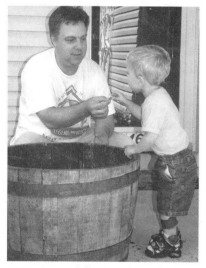

13.19

Low Sit To Stand

1. Sit on the floor cross-legged in front of a table with a rim or another piece of solid indoor or outdoor furniture with a rim or edge for your child to hold onto.
2. Have your child sit on your leg. See to it that his feet are in a good position—flat on the floor with toes pointing forward or slightly outward (photo 13.18a).
3. Encourage your child to pull to stand (photo 13.18b). If needed, assist at his hips or knees.
4. When he wants to lower himself back down, tell him to hold onto the rim well and slowly lower himself to sitting. Assist if needed.

Standing with One Arm Support

The next three activities challenge your child to further improve his balance and coordination while standing with arm support.

1. Your child stands at a table or other furniture with his feet flat on the floor and his legs shoulder-width apart.
2. As you play with your child, hold up something of interest to him and have him reach for it (photo 13.19). Doing so teaches him to balance in standing using only one hand for support.

Standing and Turning

1. Your child stands at a table with his feet flat on the floor and legs shoulder-width apart.
2. As you play with your child, hold a toy at his side and encourage him to turn and reach for it. The grab bar suctioned to the table makes the activity easier for the child in photo 13.20.

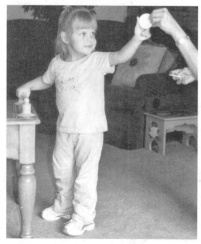

13.20

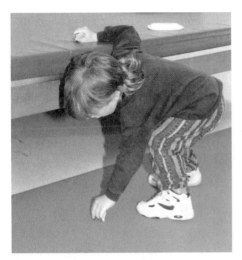

13.21

Bending Down

1. Your child stands at a table with his feet flat on the floor and shoulder-width apart.
2. Give him small toys to play with—blocks, toy animals, plastic figures, or a similar toy with small pieces. Place most of the pieces on a bench or stool at his right side and entice him to reach down and get them. If needed, help him place his right foot out to the side and stabilize it as he bends down reaching for a toy.
3. Move the stool to his left side and have him reach down to the left.
4. After a week of practice, or whenever reaching down becomes easier, try placing the toys on something lower.
5. Finally, after more practice sessions, you may drop a toy to the floor and see if he can bend all the way down to pick it up (photo 13.21).

Frequently Asked Questions

Q. *"My daughter, Emily, has a little chair with armrests just her size. It is safer than a bench. Shouldn't we use it instead of a bench?"*

A. Sure, use it. If you have a little table for it, you have a perfect set up for independent table work. But do not use the chair for sitting balance exercises. Its backrest will tempt Emily to slouch back and lift her feet off the floor. The armrests will give her something to hold onto. She will not be challenged to sit with arms free and balance.

Q. *"Chandler sits well on a little stool all by himself. But when I practice reaching with him, he becomes very insecure, hunches his shoulders, and rounds his back. Why does he do this and what should I do about it?"*

A. It seems that the reaching exercise is too difficult for Chandler. Most likely he hunches his shoulders and rounds his back to protect himself from falling backwards. Talk to your therapist about this. Together you may be able to change the exercise so it is just right for Chandler. You want him to have a good posture when he reaches.

Q. *"My son, Caleb, will come up to tall kneel but does not stay there. Why?"*

A. What you describe is very common. Caleb shows good strength by being able to come to tall kneel even briefly. What he is missing is endurance and balance. This will develop through practice and experience. Progress may be slow but you will notice it.

Q. *"Karla has braces, but even when she uses them she stands on her toes. Should I take them off because they seem not to be helping?"*

A. Before you do anything, have the physician or therapist who ordered the braces and the person who made them look at them. Most likely the braces need to be adjusted or changed. If the braces are properly fitted and Karla still tries to stand on her toes, she may be one of a few persistent children who do not want to change their ways. Even so, I recommend that you don't give up. Work closely with Karla's doctor and therapist. Together you will find a way to solve the problem.

Q. *"One of the students in my early intervention class constantly tries to pull to stand. He endangers himself and frequently falls. What should I do?"*

A. Pulling to stand is an important skill. A child with cerebral palsy needs much practice to master it. You want to guide your student's initiative, provide safety, and reward his efforts. Assign your classroom aide or volunteer to supervise and guard your student during a portion of the class time and discourage him from pulling to stand other times. With many safe practice opportunities, your student may soon improve.

14

Standing without Arm Support and Walking

When will Max walk?" "Do you think Annika will walk?" There are no other questions more often asked by parents of children with motor delays, and it is never easy to answer them. Instead, let's find out what makes it possible for children to walk on their own. Before they walk, children have to be able to do the following:

- *Walk with support* along furniture, with a walker, or held by their hands. Children who learn to walk with support have a better chance of learning to walk independently.
- *Balance in standing.* The straighter children can stand and the longer they are able to maintain their balance while standing, the sooner and better they will be able to walk.
- *Balance very briefly over one leg.* Each leg has to be strong and co-ordinated enough to support the child's body weight, so she is able to stand and balance briefly on one leg as the other leg steps forward.
- *Lower themselves from free standing to the floor with control.* Children may drop down into sitting or forward onto their extended arms. Whatever they do, if they are able to control their fall, they may not be frightened of hurting themselves. Knowing this will give them the confidence to take off and walk without support.

Which of these is most important and which should be practiced first? Let's look at how one-year-old babies start to walk. They usually walk with support for two to three months and then within one month they start to stand and walk without support. They seem to learn it all at once—standing without support, falling safely, and balancing briefly on one foot as they take their first steps.

Children with cerebral palsy try to follow the same sequence, yet it will take them much more time and effort to even partially master each skill. Balance skills especially require much training. Parents need to be patient. After the children learn to walk with arm support, some may slowly progress to walking without any support. Telling them to be brave and just walk does not help them if they do not have the necessary balance skills.

To shorten the transition from walking with support to walking without, the physical therapist may recommend early training of free standing, standing on one leg, and lowering from standing. So, instead of learning one skill after the other, a child can improve simultaneously in walking with support and balancing.

Walking with Arm Support

WALKING SIDEWAYS—CRUISING ALONG FURNITURE

Most children will take their first steps while supporting themselves at a bench or table. After pulling to stand and playing in standing, they will try to step to the side. This is not easy for them to do. They may lean heavily on their arms, come up on their toes, and accomplish only tiny steps, maybe crossing their legs in the effort. To side step, they have to shift their weight over one leg in order to take a step with the other leg. The next activities train this. Do them as directed by your child's therapist and follow his specific directions.

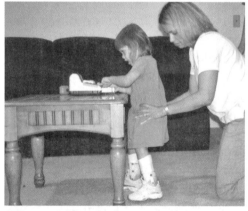

14.1

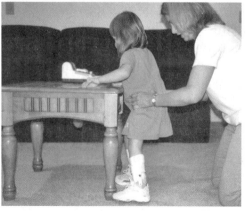

14.2

Standing and Rocking

1. Your child stands at the table supporting herself with her arms and not leaning with her trunk against it. Her feet are flat on the floor, shoulder-width apart, and her toes point forward or slightly outward.
2. Place a musical toy on the table and encourage her to rock from side to side with the music. Kneel behind her, hold her at the side of her hips, and help her move all her weight over one foot and then over to the other (photo 14.1). Say or sing: "Rock … and … rock," and give some downward pressure as you say "Rock." Repeat this for as long as your child likes.
3. Next, have her rock side-to-side without your help.

Rock and Step

1. After you have practiced rocking as described above, move the toy out of reach to the right side.
2. Tell your child: "Let's rock and then step to the toy."
3. Kneeling behind her, help her rock to the left and then step to the right side (photo 14.2). Cue her by saying: "rock … and step, rock … and step."
4. After your child has reached the toy and played with it, move it to the left side and have her step to the left.

Start out by having your child do only 2 to 4 sidesteps while you assist her. Later have her do more side steps and help her less.

Variation. If your child has difficulty stepping out to the right side, do the following:

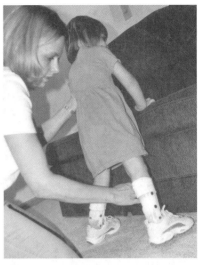

1. After you have helped her rock to the left side, support her left hip well with your left hand.
2. With your right hand, lightly push against the inner side of her right leg, helping her lift the leg out to the side as you say "step" (photo 14.3)
3. Practice similarly stepping out to the left side.

14.3

Walking Forward – One Step at a Time

This activity practices forward stepping with support and guidance. You need something stable for your child to hold onto as she walks. If your child is small you may use a stable walking toy with old nylon hose wrapped around its axles so it will not roll away. A taller child may hold onto a rung of a ladder box or a Peto walking ladder or hold onto the back of a chair. Helping your child to forward step with control is not easy. Make sure to practice the technique with the help of the physical therapist before you try it at home. Also walk with your child only a short distance this way. Longer practice may make your back ache and knees hurt. You do not want this to happen to you.

1. Your child stands holding onto the ladder with both hands. Her feet are apart, flat on the floor, and toes point forward or slightly outward.
2. Stand closely behind your child. Open your hands wide and place them firmly on the sides of her hips.
3. Ask or help your child to shift her weight over her right leg and support it well with your right hand. Slide your left hand a few inches down so your fingers rest on her upper thigh. Encourage her to step forward with her left leg while you guide her movement from her hip and upper thigh with your left hand. After she stepped, help her to push the ladder forward as much as needed.
4. Repeat and have your child step with the right leg.
5. Have her practice walking this way for a specific short distance.

Walking with a Walker

If your child is over two years of age by the time she pulls to stand, her therapist's goal will be for her to walk independently with a walker as soon as possible. For this your child will need a walker that provides her with support. There are many different types of walkers available for children with cerebral palsy. Your therapist will inform and advise you about them. Together you will decide which walker provides the right amount of support for your child and will be most functional at home, in school, and outdoors.

There are three basic types of walkers available for children with cerebral palsy: forward walkers, reverse walkers, and gait trainers.

FORWARD WALKERS

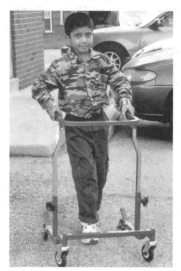

14.4

Forward walkers have vertical or horizontal handlebars to hold onto (photo 14.4). The children hold onto them and push the walker in front as they walk. Forward walkers are economically priced and easy to use. The children learn to stand up to them from chair sitting and to lower themselves to chair sitting or to the floor when they no longer want to walk. A forward walker is most useful for a child who needs just balance support (photo 14.4). If the child needs to lean onto her arms when she stands and steps, the walker has serious drawbacks. It encourages children to bend at the hip and lean forward with their trunk. This position will reinforce the abnormal scissoring pattern of a child who tends to walk on forefeet and toes.

REVERSE WALKERS

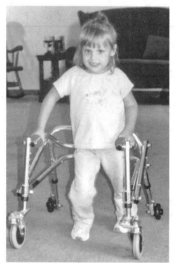

14.5

The reverse walker discourages toe walking. It has a horizontal U-shaped bar that gives hand support at the sides, as well as back protection (photo 14.5). Instead of pushing it, a child pulls it along as she walks. The design of the walker provides safety against a backwards fall. It encourages children to stand tall and walk without leaning forward or crouching. The walker is sturdy, not prone to tipping, fairly easy to steer, and the basic model folds flat. With some training, a child may learn to stand up to the walker and lower herself to the floor—thus becoming fully independent with it.

Children who have good strength and control of the muscles of both arms usually do well with a reverse walker. If your child has been pushing to hands and knees and crawling, this type of walker may be recommended for her. The therapist will train your child to walk with the walker, and, as soon as possible, show you how to use it at home. Soon, standing up to the walker and lowering to the floor will become part of your child's training. The following activities are examples of how to do this. Use them as directed by your therapist.

Pulling to Stand at a Reverse Walker

1. Encourage your child to crawl to the walker, reach up, place her hands on the sidebars, and pull to tall kneel (photo 14.6a).
2. Stabilize the walker for her and encourage her to stand up via half-kneel or as shown in photo 14.6b. She will be facing the bar in the back of the walker and needs to turn around before walking with the walker. (See next activity.)

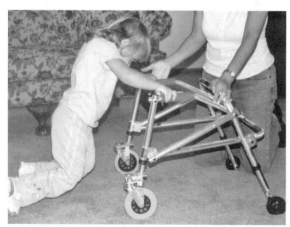

14.6a

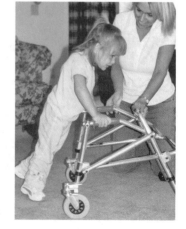

14.6b

Turning Around in the Walker

1. Stabilize the walker for your child.
2. Ask her to stand tall, step into the walker with her left foot, move her right hand over to the back bar or left sidebar (photo 14.7), and bring her right foot forward and around.
3. Have her take baby steps to adjust her feet.
4. Have her adjust her hands. When she is ready, have her turn her trunk and reach with her left hand over to the other sidebar.
5. Some more baby steps to the left, and she will stand facing forward, ready to walk with the walker.

Do the activity in the opposite direction if turning clockwise is easier for her.

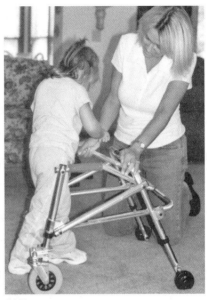

14.7

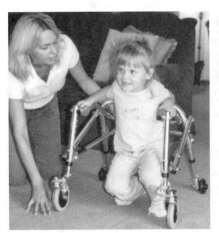

14.8a

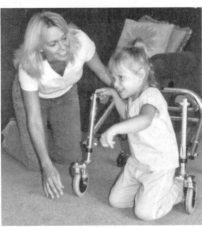

14.8b

Lowering from the Walker to the Floor

1. Stabilize the walker for your child.
2. Ask her to stand tall and put all her weight on her arms.
3. With your help as needed, have her kick one foot back, bend the other knee, bend her elbows, lower herself into half-kneel (photo 14.8a), and then kneel on the floor.
4. Now she is ready to let go of the walker (photo 14.8b), catch herself with her arms on the floor, and crawl away.

GAIT TRAINERS

Children who do not have good control over their arm and shoulder muscles will need more support than the reverse walker provides. If your child is unable to push to a hand and knee position or crawl on all fours, walking in a reverse walker would be unsafe.

The gait trainer is the walker of choice for children whose arms and legs are seriously affected by cerebral palsy (photo 14.9). Gait trainers have the support and safety features these children need. They have chest support, which will hold the child in an upright position. With the chest support secured, even a child who cannot fully bear weight over her legs may stand and take steps. A saddle or sling seat is another feature most gait trainers have. These seats allow the child to straddle sit if her legs buckle.

Gait trainers are more expensive than other walkers. They roll easily, but may be difficult to steer for the child who uses it. Transfers in and out of a gait trainer may pose a problem. Initially, a child may need the assistance of one or two persons. However, these walkers provide the opportunity to stand and take steps for children who otherwise would not have it.

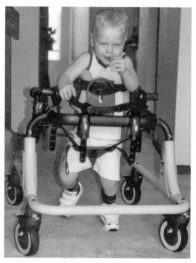

Gait trainers are bulky and difficult to transport. The exception is the Pacer Gait Trainer. Its frame folds for transport in the trunk of the car.

After the child is able to take steps fully supported, she is taught to hold onto the bars of the walker and stand or step with less chest support. The goal will be that eventually the child walks without chest support.

14.9

Improving the Way Your Child Walks with a Walker

The better your child walks with a walker, the easier it is for her, and the more she will walk. Ankle braces (AFOs) will help her to place her feet flat on the floor. Stepping forward without turning her legs in, crossing over the other foot, or stumbling may take time. Practicing and learning a variety of stepping and walking skills will help your child to gain more control over her leg movements. Mastering sidestepping along furniture, turning around a corner while holding on, and stair walking with assistance will improve her strength and coordination. All of this will help her to walk better.

Strong arms will also help her to walk better with a walker. You may be surprised to hear this and wonder why. Holding onto the walker with strong arms will make your child feel safe. If she can rely on her arms she won't be afraid of falling each time her legs tangle up and cause her to stumble. Her strong arms will hold her up, give her time to fix her feet, and continue on.

As your child improves she may start to like to walk with her walker anywhere. You are glad about it, but you may also worry. Your child may walk her own way and not how you and her therapist want her to walk. She may turn one foot in, not put her heels down, walk too fast, run into things, and so on. What should parents do about this? Tell their child she walks sloppily, to watch her steps, and to slow down? Walking is a very personal thing. You wouldn't want to be criticized about the way you walk, would you? The same is true for your child. She worked hard to be able to walk with a walker. She does not want to be told she walks sloppily. And yet it may be good for her to improve the way she walks. Her walking pattern may stress her hip or knee joints if she walks like this for many years. What to do? The following is a suggestion on how to train your child to walk better.

Walking with Guidance

1. Choose a specific time and a specific distance for your child to walk with you each day.

2. Have her stand in her walker with feet apart, flat on the floor, and toes pointing forward or slightly outward.

3. Choose a specific problem you want her to fix, such as placing her right foot more forward. Ask her to walk very slowly and do her best to place her foot better. Walk next to her. Help her with your words. As she readies to step with her right foot you say "step forward." You may have her say it with you.

4. Praise her whenever she succeeds in placing her foot better.

5. Make the daily good walking trip a game. Count each good step, write down the total as her score for the day, and post it on the refrigerator.

Walking with Reduced Support

The next exercises train children to walk with less support than a walker provides. Your therapist may recommend them after your child has learned to walk well with a walker or if she believes that your child is capable of walking independently without using a walker first. Whatever the case, please follow your therapist's instructions when using these activities.

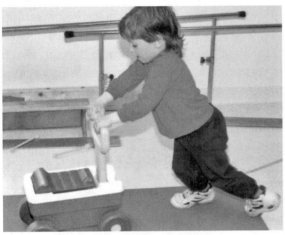

14.10

Walking with a Toy Cart

1. Your child stands with feet flat on the floor, shoulder-width apart, and toes pointing forward or slightly outward.

2. Have your child hold onto a toy cart as shown in photo 14.10, a toy shopping cart, or another suitable walking toy.

3. Secure the cart for her as you encourage her to step forward. After a few steps, see if she can walk with the cart on her own.

If the cart rolls too fast, causing her to trip and fall, slow it by wrapping nylon hose around the axles. Encourage your child to keep her feet apart. If she is unable to do so, discontinue the activity.

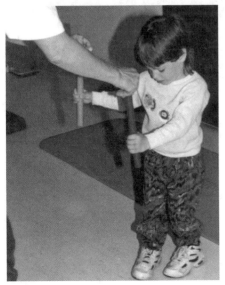

14.11

Walking with Sticks

1. Your child stands with feet flat on the floor, shoulder-width apart, and toes pointing forward or slightly outward.

2. Use the same sticks you used in "Knee Walking with Sticks" or cut a broomstick in half. Stand in front of your child holding the sticks vertically in front of her so that she can grasp them at waist-level or slightly above.

3. As your child grasps the sticks, encourage her to slowly walk with you (photo 14.11). You may cue her by saying: "step and step and step…." If necessary, remind her not to turn her feet in.

If your child is able to walk with you, make walking with sticks a daily routine and increase the distance walked.

Walking with a Hoop

1. Your child stands with feet flat on the floor, shoulder-width apart, and toes pointing forward or slightly outward.
2. Stand in front of your child, and hold a hoop out so she can grasp it at waist level with both hands.
3. Encourage her to hold onto the hoop and walk with you (photo 14.12). Remind her not to turn her feet in. Walk with her as long as she likes.

Variation. If your child needs more support, try the following. Stand behind your child and let your child stand inside the hoop, hold on to it, and walk forward with you.

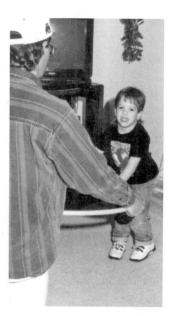

14.12

Walking with Crutches

When your child is three years or older, walks well with a walker, but is not ready to walk independently your physical therapist may recommend forearm crutches. In the past, parents often frowned upon crutch walking. Yet, today crutches are becoming more acceptable. Pediatric supply companies sell nice, sleek forearm crutches in various colors. Still, you may wonder why crutch walking is an advantage for your child. "Don't they provide much less support?" you wonder. It is true that a walker provides sturdier support than crutches. Your child needs good shoulder and arm strength and coordination to walk with crutches. Once a child has learned to walk with them and feels secure with crutches, she will prefer them to a walker. Crutches allow her to walk fast, make tight turns, get around in a small space, go through narrow doorways, walk stairs, and do curbs with ease. A child who is used to crutches will feel that walking with a walker is slow and cumbersome.

Walking with crutches is best trained by a physical therapist. Safety is important initially. The physical therapist most likely will use a gait belt during crutch training. There are no crutch training home instructions in this book. They are available elsewhere if your physical therapist wants to give them to you (Martin, 1998).

Standing without Arm Support

Standing balance training includes standing with straight and bent knees, standing, and stooping, as well as moving in and out of standing without support. It is a continuation of the standing balance activities practiced previously with arm support. It is best to use them daily during the months your child is learning to walk with support and is getting ready for independent walking.

When children balance in standing, the muscles of their lower legs, feet, and toes have to work very hard. These are usually very weak and may be spastic in children with cerebral palsy. If your child has high muscle tone and tends to stand on her toes, loosen and stretch her ankle and foot muscles with these activities described in Chapter 5:

● *Ankle Rolls*
● *Calf Muscle Stretch in Deep Squatting*

Your therapist may recommend that you do them before practicing standing balance with your child. When working on the following exercises, your child should wear tennis shoes or flexible braces, or be barefoot, but should not wear rigid braces or socks alone. These exercises cannot be done with rigid braces because they do not allow the ankle to bend, and socks are too slippery.

Use the balance activities as directed by your child's therapist and follow any specific directions given.

Your Child Stands between Your Legs

1. Sit on the edge of a chair and have your child stand between your legs, holding onto them and facing you.
2. Help your child to stand with feet flat on the floor, shoulder-width apart, and toes pointing forward or slightly turned outward.
3. Look at a book together. Have your child point to pictures, turn pages (thereby taking one or both hands off your leg), and eventually even hold the book and stand with no hand support. Or hold a toy and encourage your child to take her hands off your legs and play with it, finally holding the toy by herself (and standing free).
4. Guard your child well and protect her from falling. Whenever your child loses her good leg position, help her to come back to it.

Variation. If your child tends to turn her feet inward and come up on her toes, take your shoes off and place your feet over her feet (photo 14.13). The weight of your feet will help your child to keep her feet flat on the floor, provide some stability, and make it easier for her to stand without arm support.

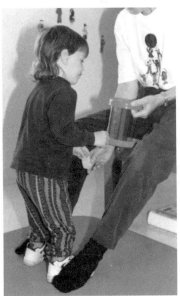

14.13

Your Child Stands between Your Legs and Bends Down

After your child is comfortable standing and playing without holding on to you for a minute or more, try the following.

1. Play as before, but now occasionally hold something low so your child has to bend down as she reaches for it (photo 14.14).
2. Observe her legs and remind her not to press her knees together as she bends down. If she loses her correct foot position, wait for her to regain her balance and "fix her feet."

Pushing to Stand and Coming Down

After your child has learned to bend and then straighten her legs again without falling, she is ready to try this activity. It will teach her to rise to standing and to safely lower herself from standing. This will boost her self-confidence and make her less fearful of falling. Use the activity as directed by your child's therapist.

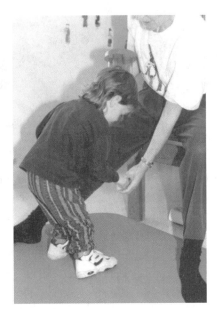

14.14

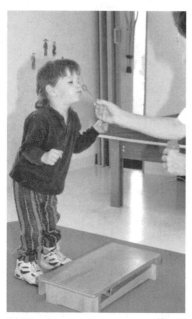

14.15

1. Place a bench or heavy box in the middle of the room away from furniture.
2. Ask your child to crawl to it and put her hands on the box. Help her place her feet on the floor about shoulder-width apart (most likely her heels will not touch the floor).
3. Now, from in front of her, ask her to rise to standing. (A high bench or box will make this easier and a low bench more difficult.)
4. Encourage her to blow bubbles while she stands as long as possible (photo 14.15). As soon as she becomes unsteady, encourage her to bend at the hip and support herself with her arms on the bench.

Another time when she rises to standing, together you can look at a sheet of nice stickers or Colorforms. Have her talk about them, choose one, take it, bend down, and arrange one sticker after another on the box.

Variation. If your child has difficulties keeping her feet flat on the floor, see if adding some weight might help. Put soft wrist or ankle weights with Velcro closures loosely around your child's ankles. They will weight your child's heels down, making it easier to stand with firmly planted feet.

Standing in Front of a Wall

When standing in front of a bench, your child will lean slightly forward with her trunk. This helps prevent a backwards fall and allows her to quickly catch herself with her arms. It is a good initial standing posture. But you also want your child to stand and balance with a straight posture. This may be safely practiced as described below.

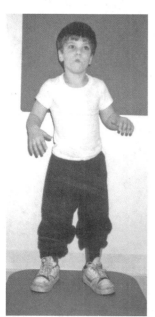

14.16

1. Help your child to stand straight with her back against a wall. Stand in front of her so she can support herself well on your outstretched forearms.
2. Ask your child to step a few inches away from the wall and stand with a nice straight posture—hips and knees straight, feet flat, shoulder-width apart, and toes pointing forward or slightly outward.
3. Challenge her to take her hands off your arms and stand by herself. If she can do this, position yourself at her side and guard her well without touching her.
4. Together count how long she can stand by herself. When she becomes unsteady, have her regain her balance by bending her hips slightly and resting her bottom against the wall.
5. Practice the activity until your child does it consistently well. Now you may have her practice on her own like the child in photo 14.16.

Note: Be a good observer. Always quickly and calmly support your child when she is in danger of falling. During early independent standing balance exercises, children may be very fearful of falling. Even a fall that does not hurt may make them overly cautious and reluctant to try the same activity again. On the other hand, children will thrive and gain confidence from safe, successful balance experiences.

Pushing to Stand from the Floor

1. Ask your child to crawl to the middle of the room away from any furniture.
2. Encourage her to place her feet on the floor about shoulder-width apart (most likely his heels will not touch the floor), straighten her legs as much as possible, and rise to standing.

3. During initial practices you may help her to place her feet in the correct position. As your child improves, have her do it on her own.

Variation. If your child cannot stand up by pushing up from the floor, have her push up from a low bench or stepping stool (photo 14.17). As she improves place something lower such as a telephone book on the floor. Continue to practice with her until she can stand up from the floor.

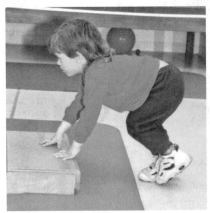

14.17

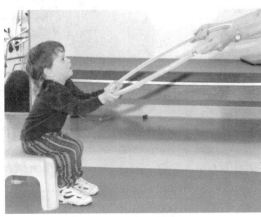

14.18a

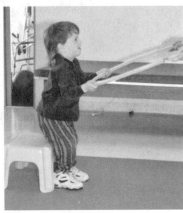

14.18b

Standing Up and Sitting Down Holding onto a Hoop

This activity and the two following activities train your child to stand up from sitting and sit down with control. Use them as directed by your therapist.

1. Have your child sit on a bench or stool with her feet placed comfortably on the floor. Her knees are apart and her toes point forward.
2. Stand in front of your child with a hoop. Ask her to hold onto the hoop with both hands (photo 14.18a), lean her trunk forward—nose over toes—and stand up (14.18b). Remind her not to press her legs together as she comes up.
3. Next have her sit back down slowly and softly.

Try to do several repetitions. A reward after five up and downs will make it more fun for your child.

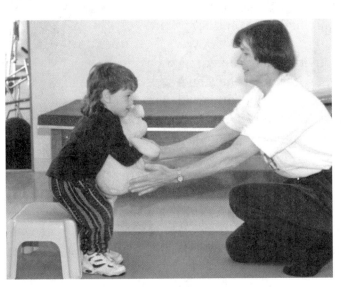

14.19

Standing Up and Sitting Down with Minimal Help

1. Have your child sit as before and have her hug her favorite stuffed toy.
2. Ask her to lean forward and have piggy stand up with her (photo 14.19). If needed, help her briefly and tell her not to push her knees together.
3. Later have her sit down slowly and softly.
4. Ask, "Is there another animal you want to bring up?" As she holds different things, have her come up and sit down as often as she is willing to play the game.

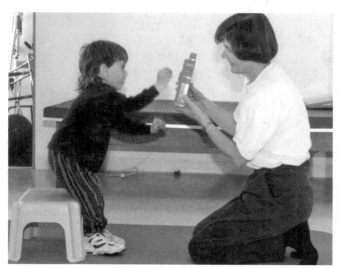
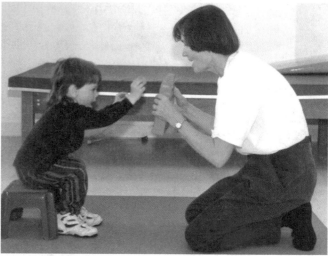

14.20a
14.20b

Standing Up and Sitting Down without Help

Even after your child is able to stand up without assistance, more practice will be helpful. It will further improve her coordination and leg strength. You will notice that she will come up with more ease and sit down with more control.

1. Choose a play activity your child likes that she can play in sitting or standing. Placing chips into a music box or play money into a small cash register may be fun.
2. Hold the toy chest-high for play in standing (photo 14.20a) and hold it low for play in sitting (photo 14.20b). Have her stand up and sit down with each turn.
3. If your child loses her good foot or leg position—her feet turn in or her knees touch—have her "fix her feet" and then continue.

Standing and Reaching Up

As your child's standing balance improves, your therapist may recommend the next two activities.

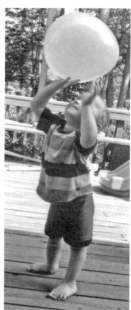

1. Help your child to stand up in the middle of the room away from any furniture or other things she could fall and hurt herself on. Ask her to place her feet flat on the floor, shoulder-width apart, and toes pointing forward or slightly outward.
2. Engage her in a play activity and have her reach up with either hand and later with both. For instance, you may ask her to reach up high with both arms and then gently drop a balloon into her hands (photo 14.21).

This activity requires concentration. Stop as soon as you notice that your child is getting tired.

Playing Ball

1. Ask your child to stand up in the middle of the room away from furniture or any clutter.

14.21

2. Have her stand with her feet flat on the floor, shoulder-width apart, and toes pointing forward or slightly outward.

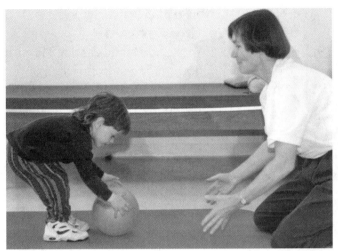

14.22a

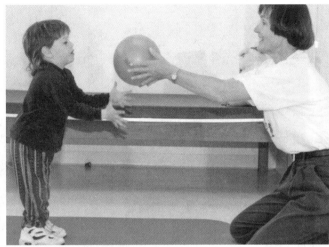

14.22b

3. Gently roll a ball toward her feet and encourage her to slowly bend down, pick it up (photo 14.22a), and hand it to you.

4. Next ask her to hold her arms out. Say, "Good catch" as you drop and later throw the ball into her hands (photo 14.22b). "Now toss the ball to me."

Gentle ball play is fun and will develop your child's balance. Keep it as simple as possible. If she loses her good foot position, pause and wait for her to "fix her feet" before you continue.

Assisted Standing on One Leg

As you walk, your left leg supports your body weight when your right leg swings forward. As you put the right foot down, both legs support your weight. Then your left leg swings forward and your right leg carries your weight until you set your left foot down and both legs support your weight. This cycle is repeated over and over as you walk. Bearing all body weight on one leg is an essential component of walking without arm support.

When children walk with a walker or forearm crutches, they bear part of their weight with their arms. Instead of bearing all their weight on one leg as they step forward, they distribute it on the leg and their arms.

You might have experienced this yourself if you hurt one leg and your doctor ordered you to walk with crutches while your injury healed. Walking with crutches without putting weight on one leg was possible but cumbersome and tiring for your hands, arms, and shoulders. You were relieved when you were allowed to put some weight on the injured foot. Now crutch walking was easier.

Similarly, the more weight children can bear on either leg, the easier it is for them to walk with a walker or crutches and to progress to walking without an assistive device. Physical therapists recommend that parents practice one leg standing with their children as early as possible. They can do this by incorporating one leg standing into their children's dressing routine. This will provide a brief but consistent exercise time and also trains an independent dressing skill.

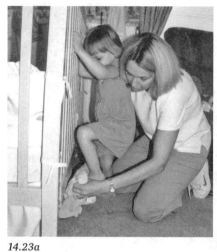

14.23a

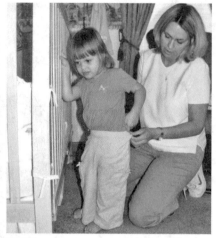

14.23b

One Foot Standing While Getting Dressed

1. Your child stands and holds with both hands onto the slats of the crib, the edge of the playpen, a wall bar, or a standing ladder.
2. Kneel behind her and support her as much as needed. Ask her to lift one leg at a time while you pull the pants legs over her feet (photo 14.23a).
3. Then have her stand tall on both legs while you pull her pants up (photo 14.23b).

4. Reverse the process when you help her to take off her pants.

Variation A. If your child does well, have her stand holding on without your support. Hold the pant leg open and ask her to lift her leg and put her foot through it.

Variation B. After you have helped her to pull the pant legs over her feet, see if she can stand holding onto the wall bar with one hand and help you pull her pants up with her other hand. Similarly, have her practice taking her pants off.

Discontinue the one leg standing practice during dressing time when your child is ready to put her pants on all by herself. Teach her to sit and pull her pants over her feet. Then have her stand up, hold onto the wall bar with one hand, and pull her pants up with the other hand.

For more one leg standing practice, use the exercises described in the next chapter.

Extra Standing Time for the Weaker Leg

Most children with cerebral palsy have a marked difference between their legs. Usually one is stronger, more coordinated, and shows better balance than the other. This is especially true for children with hemiplegia. Naturally, children will favor the less affected leg and mostly stand on it. This may work for standing but not for walking. When a child tries to walk and one leg is too weak to support her weight or too uncoordinated to balance over it, she is unable to walk safely without an assistive device.

To improve the strength and coordination of the weaker leg, children are asked to place their stronger leg on a stool and stand on their weaker leg (this is called half-standing). Now the muscles of the weaker leg have to do the work to keep the child standing. As children play in half-standing, they will move slightly and shift their weight. This will challenge the child's stance and lead to improvement of the coordination and balance responses of the weaker leg.

Exercises in half-standing may be used to prepare children for walking or to improve the gait of children who are already walking independently. Half-standing with straight knee and hip of the standing leg and good heel-to-floor contact also stretches tight calf muscles and trains full weight bearing through the straight knee. Depending on your child's capability and the training objectives, her therapist will choose the best-suited half-standing position and determine the height of the stool used.

You may find that the exercises in half-standing are difficult for your child at first. She may easily lose her balance. In the beginning, support her well. As you sit or kneel at her side, wrap your arm around her waist or hips until she stands solidly. Then move your arm a few inches away so you are no longer touching her, but be ready to support her again as needed. Also be a good observer. Your child may "cheat" when she half-stands. Instead of standing mostly on the straight leg, she may lean onto her bent leg. This defeats the purpose of the exercise and increases the danger of falling.

It will take some time for you and your child to be comfortable with half-standing activities. Once learned, they will be easy, even relaxing. They will allow for many different play situations, and most of all, they are very beneficial for your child, especially if she has hemiplegic cerebral palsy.

Use the exercises as directed by your child's therapist and follow any specific recommendations given.

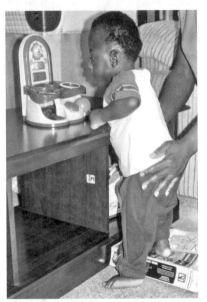

Half-Standing at Furniture

1. Have your child stand at a table or other furniture of good height.
2. Have her stand on her weaker leg and place her stronger leg on a stool or a thick phone book (photo 14.24). The foot and the knee are pointing forward. If initially your child cannot prevent the knee from turning in, hold the knee in the right position. Later reduce your support.
3. Place her favorite toys on a table or other furniture of a good height in front of her and encourage her to play with them.
4. Initially support your child well at the hips and make sure that her foot is flat on the floor with toes pointing forward or slightly outward.
5. Take your hands off her hips, have her stand without your support, and guard her well.

Discontinue the activity if her standing leg is bent and her other knee points inward.

14.24

Standing on the Weaker Leg

1. Sit on the edge of a chair and have your child stand between your legs facing you with her stronger leg placed on a stool. This way most of her weight is on her weaker leg. If needed, let her hold onto you for support.
2. Look at interesting picture books to make the activity enjoyable for both of you.

Variation A. If your child's bent knee turns inward, support it so it points forward (photo 14.25a).

Variation B. If your child bends the knee of the leg she stands on, try to brace it with your leg. Discontinue the activity if she cannot straighten the knee with your help at least part of the time.

Variation C. If your child does well, have her try to do the activity without any support. For instance have her look at a pop-up book. Let her turn the pages, pull the tab,

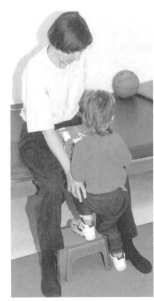

14.25a

etc. When she plays with a shape drum, have her hold the drum with one hand and reach for the shape with the other. Also have her practice reaching up and bending down (14.25b).

Progress with Standing Balance

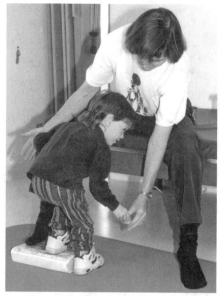

14.25b

Standing balance takes much work to achieve. *It is not a matter of working on it several days or weeks, but daily practice of maybe several months.* "I don't have that much time," you might protest. Think about it again. How much time do you spend each day reading to or playing with your child? Most likely it is more than half an hour. This is the time you can use for balance training. Use books or toys your child likes for the standing balance activities—soon you and your child will feel like you're playing together instead of working. Yet, work is being done.

Progress will be slow but will occur. Watch for the little changes. The first week, your child may lose the correct foot position within 10 seconds, the next week she may stand nicely and balance up to 20 seconds, then for 25 seconds and so on. Feeling more secure, your child may start to move more in standing. But when she does so, she becomes more likely to lose her good leg position. You may feel defeated because the tendency to turn the legs inward will not go away. Don't quit. The tendency to turn the legs in may never totally disappear but will happen less often, become less disruptive, and most of all will not keep her from walking with feet flat.

Your child has already learned to stand very still. Now she is learning to control her posture and balance while her body moves. Each time she does something new—reaching up, bending down, throwing a ball—she will start out very unsteady and show a poor posture. Then, slowly her posture and balance will improve. All this work will pay off when your child tries to walk. The better her standing balance is, the better her chances are for independent walking without a walker or crutches.

Progress with half-standing may be even more subtle and more difficult to detect. Yet even a slight improvement of the weaker leg will make a difference. Your child may fall less, walk faster, become able to kick a ball—all because her more affected leg has improved in coordination and balance.

Strength and Quick Action

Good muscle strength always helps, but being able to move fast and quickly tighten your muscles is also important. When walking, you lift your foot, move it forward, and then put it down. Muscles that keep your knee straight have to work immediately; otherwise you could not stand on the leg and take another step. In fact, our leg muscles do not have to be very strong. (Of course, they need to be strong enough to hold us up.) As long as the muscles do the right thing, at the right time, and at the right speed, we can walk fine.

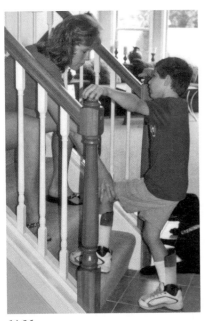

14.26

These exercises train quick stepping and standing. They may be used to get your child ready for independent walking or to improve the way she walks. Use the exercises if recommended by your child's therapist and follow any specific instructions given.

Quick Step Up and Down

This exercise works best on stairs.
1. You sit on the third or fourth step facing your child.
2. Have your child hold onto the banister with her hands and place her left foot on the first step. Make sure her foot and knee point forward.
3. Brace her left knee with your right hand (photo 14.26), preventing it from turning inward while she quickly steps up onto the first step with her right leg. Pause.
4. Ask her to quickly step down with the right leg. Pause.
5. Repeat 10 times.
6. Repeat 10 times with the opposite leg.

Quick Step-Down

1. Start with your child standing on the first step, facing downstairs, holding onto the banister with her hands and ready to step down.
2. Sit in a chair in front of your child, bracing her left knee with your right hand.
3. Ask her to quickly step down with her right foot (photo 14.27). Pause.
4. Then have her bring her right foot back up. Repeat 10 times.
5. Repeat the exercise 10 times with the other leg.

Note: These are real exercises—no play at all. A school-age child may be agreeable to do them, but a two-year-old child may not. It will help to have a nice reward for her after she completes a set of exercises.

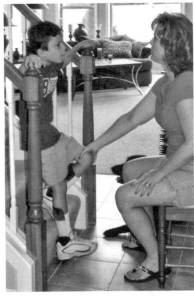

14.27

Walking

"Stand up, Camdon," his mother coaxes. "Show Mrs. Martin what you can do." Three-year-old Camdon pushes up from the floor and rises to standing. He does it slowly and carefully. "That's right, put your heel down. Look how nicely you are standing!" Mom is pleased. Camdon has managed to stand up without any help and stands with his feet firmly planted on the ground and a nice posture. But there are more surprises for the therapist. "Are you ready?" Mom asks and lightly tosses a ball to him. Camdon sways as he catches the ball. For a brief moment it looks as if he may lose his balance. But it passes and he does not fall. "You are doing great," his mother beams. Standing confidently again, Camdon half throws and half drops the ball back to his mother.

Catching it, she turns to the therapist: "Isn't he doing well? He learned it this week." The therapist is truly amazed. None of her patients who had not yet begun to walk without support had ever done anything like this.

Camdon still struggles when walking with a walker. Tightly holding onto the walker, his body leans forward and his legs drag behind. He wants to step fast but his legs are not cooperating. They cross over and his heels do not touch the floor. When Camdon walks with his mother, he does a better job. She slows him down, asks him to watch his feet, and place each foot flat on the floor without crossing over. When he walks this way, his body sways from side to side and he firmly holds onto his mother's hands.

Having observed him walk this way, the therapist has been doubtful that Camdon would be able to walk without support any time soon. But now watching him stand up and play ball in standing, she becomes much more hopeful. Camdon seems to sense when he stands well, knows when his balance is threatened, and can regain a good standing position when his balance is mildly challenged. If he loses his balance, he does not fall uncontrolled but crouches and gently drops to the side.

Camdon is no longer afraid to stand. He enjoys it. Each week his standing posture becomes a little surer. A few weeks later, at the start of Camdon's session, the mother and the therapist talk and decide to try something new. After Camdon stands up, the therapist places a therapy roll upright in front of him, about a foot out of his reach (photo 14.28). She puts a toy animal on top of the roll. "Take a step and get the horse, Camdon," Mom encourages. The therapy roll looks substantial but would topple over if Camdon tried to take a big step and lunged for it. Camdon plays it safe. He takes a small step with his right foot and then with his left foot. Almost close enough, he stops to regain his balance. With brief help from the therapist, he succeeds. Two more steps and he lightly touches the roll, reaches for the toy and regains his standing balance without help. What a success!

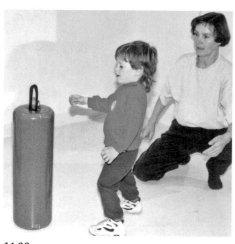

14.28

With little pauses in between, Camdon practices the same activity again and again. Regaining his standing balance after one or two steps becomes easier. Walking further does not yet work out. A week later, however, he manages to walk four steps in a row, stop, and regain his balance without any help. This is the way Camdon is learning to walk and make progress—one small step at a time.

"Will my child start to walk the way Camdon did?" you wonder. Most likely not; each child is unique. Before you decide to help your child to walk on her own, you must find out if she can walk fast or if she needs to take very slow steps.

One-year-old children usually choose a fast start. When they take off on their own, they do not take measured, slow steps, but almost run. They step/step/step/step, fall down, get up, step/step/step/step/step, hold on, and so on.

Children who begin to walk when they are two years or older tend to walk slower and will be more careful to avoid a fall. Being taller, dropping onto their bottom as one-year-olds may do is uncomfortable for them. They may plan ahead and try to hold on to something when they fear that they may lose their balance.

Watch your child walk with a walker or when you hold her hands. Many children with cerebral palsy lose control when they walk fast. Their legs turn inward and they trip and fall. At a slow speed, this is less likely to happen. Consequently, they have to start walking at a very slow speed. This poses a problem. Walking at a slow speed requires better balance than walking fast, because when you are walking slowly the time spent on just one foot is longer and the momentum of the movement does not help you.

If your child needs to walk slowly in order to control her leg movements, it is important that you get a feel for her situation. Understanding how she needs to walk will help you work together with her therapist so your child can progress toward this important goal. Pretend you have to walk over a narrow bridge spanning a swift creek. Would you rather cross it quickly or very slowly? Walking fast may cause you to stumble and fall into the water. So you have to play it safe and walk slowly. This is similar to the situation many children with cerebral palsy face. Walking slowly is their only option.

If your child has low muscle tone or a milder form of cerebral palsy, her therapist may advise you that there is no need to slow your child down. Instead she may recommend that your child choose her own walking speed and the distance she dares to walk on her own.

The subsequent activities practice slow controlled walking, first with minimal arm support and then without. Use them if recommended by your physical therapist and follow any specific instructions given.

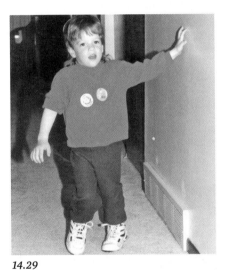

14.29

Walking with One Hand against a Wall

1. Have your child stand at a 90-degree angle to a wall, close enough to touch it, with her feet shoulder-width apart and toes pointing forward or slightly outward.
2. Stand a few feet in front of her and encourage her to walk toward you while bracing herself with one hand against the wall (photo 14.29). Remind her to walk slowly and not point her feet inward. If she does well, have her walk increasingly longer distances.
3. Repeat in the opposite direction.

Variation. If the activity is too difficult for your child, give her more support. Walk besides her, holding a short stick, and have her hold onto it with her free hand.

Repeat in the opposite direction.

Green Light – Red Light

Initially, Camdon could only walk a couple of steps and then had to stop to regain his balance. Practicing stopping and starting will help children gain balance control.

1. Your child stands as before, supporting herself with one hand against the wall and the other hand holding onto a stick you hold.
2. Ask her to play green light – go, red light – stop with you. Say: "Green Light" and walk side by side a few steps.
3. Next say: "Red Light." You both stop and you let her hold the stick by herself. This will challenge her to regain her standing balance independently.
4. Hold onto the stick again when she is ready for "Green Light" and more walking side by side.

Practice as long as your child is interested. For variety, let her be the one who says "Red Light" or "Green Light."

Variation. After your child does well with the activity, see if she can walk with you holding onto the stick with one hand and only lightly touching the wall with the fingers of the other hand. During red light have her hold the stick by herself and stand with just her fingers at the wall for support.

Your Child Walks Slowly toward You

If your child is able to control a fall, use this suggestion to encourage her to take independent steps. Practice it as directed by your child's therapist.

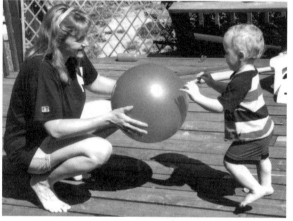

14.30

1. Ask your child to stand on her own with feet flat, shoulder-width apart, and toes pointing forward or slightly turned outward.
2. Stand or squat about one to two feet out of her reach and hold a ball with both hands (photo 14.30).
3. Tell her: "Slowly step and step and get the ball." Wait for your child to come to you. You may reassure her with your voice but do not try to give support. Your stretched out hand will not be helpful. It will make your child think about holding on instead of concentrating on maintaining her balance.
4. If your child succeeds, she deserves a hug and a short break before you have her try again.

Walking Between Two Ropes

This exercise may help a child who is able to place her feet well and appears to be ready to walk on her own. Walking between ropes will provide minimal support, but will be easier than walking entirely unassisted. It teaches what free walking is all about.

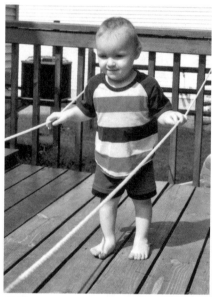

14.31

1. Attach two ropes to solid pieces of furniture. Make them parallel at the height and width just right for your child. When children first walk, they hold their arms out to keep their balance. The ropes should be where your child would hold her hands if she walked on her own.
2. Have your child walk between the ropes (photo 14.31).

TYPICAL METHODS OF ENCOURAGING WALKING

There are time-honored and popular ways parents encourage their children to walk, including the three listed below. How helpful are they for children with cerebral palsy?

Walking from One Person to Another

Samantha stands with Mom. Dad is a few feet away, stretches his arms out, and calls: "Sammy, come to Daddy!" Sammy will take a few quick steps and fall into Dad's arm. This is fun. Later Dad will discourage Sammy from lunging forward. He will call her to come and not stretch his arms out. He will hug her after she has walked all the way to him.

This activity will not help a child who needs to walk slowly in order to control each step and keep her balance.

Walking with and Then without Support

Sammy holds onto Mom's finger and walks with her. After several steps, Mom pulls her finger out of Sammy's hand and has Sammy walk on her own.

Most likely this technique will not help a child with cerebral palsy. If you want to try it nevertheless, *make sure that your child knows when she is no longer supported.* The awareness of being on her own will help your child to concentrate and deal with any balance threat as best she can. If your child believes she is protected from a fall by you, but is not, she may get hurt if she falls unexpectedly.

Protecting Your Child from Falling by Holding onto His Clothing

Holding onto Sammy's collar, her mother walks with her. After several steps, she lets go of it and has Sammy continue on her own.

This does not help most beginning walkers with cerebral palsy because in order to keep their balance, the children sway from side to side. Holding onto their clothing will interfere with this.

You may use this technique to provide safety when your child climbs onto furniture or playground equipment.

Ready for Walking

The following are general recommendations for children ready to walk:

A Play Corner for Standing and Stepping

- With several pieces of furniture, create an area where it is fun for your child to stand and play (photos 14.32a, b, c).
- Use child-size play kitchen furniture, a table, heavy large boxes, or whatever you can find that is the right height to encourage your child to play while standing.
- Leave spaces between the furniture to encourage your child to move about with minimal arm support or to take an independent step.

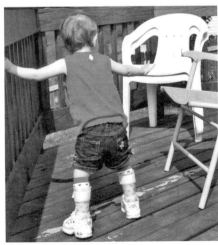

14.32a

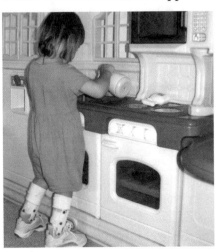

14.32b

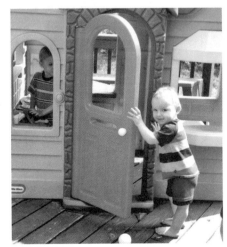

14.32c

Days Filled with Walking

- Keep your child physically fit and ready for those first independent steps with lots of standing and walking with support.
- Instead of pushing her in a stroller or carrying her, have her walk with you. If she goes to preschool or daycare, talk to her teachers or care provider about ways that can encourage her to walk.
- On weekends, keep the time your child sits in a car, rides in a shopping cart, or watches TV or videos at an absolute minimum. A child who spends most of her day sitting is not likely to start independent walking.

Frequently Asked Questions

Q. *"Chelsea does not like to stand. She used to when she was little. But now when I try to get her to stand between my legs, she drops to the floor and crawls away. What should I do?"*
A. What you describe happens frequently. While small children usually like to stand, older preschool children may rather play on the floor. Talk to Chelsea's therapist about this. The therapist may recommend that Chelsea wear knee immobilizers when she stands. It will make standing easier for her and she may like it better. As her attitude improves, she may later also stand without the immobilizers.

Q. *"Tom has a hemiparesis. His right leg is thinner and half an inch shorter than his left leg. I can't believe that half-standing exercises will make any difference. His hemiparesis will not go away."*
A. It is true that half-standing will not cure Tom's leg. No exercise in this book or otherwise will cure cerebral palsy. The exercises will train Tom's muscles and may improve his functional skills. If you do 15 minutes of half-standing with Tom daily for several weeks, you may notice that his ability to stand on the right leg improves. For instance, he may then be able to stand on his right leg while he kicks a ball with the left leg.

Q. *"Our son's therapist told us not to practice walking with him. She said that Will would walk when he was ready, and Will did start to walk on his own. Why do you give so much advice concerning walking?"*
A. Children with cerebral palsy have different capabilities. Your therapist knew Will and gave you good advice. Other children with cerebral palsy benefit from gait training. The walking exercises are for these children and should be done as directed by their therapists.

Q. *"When Aaron stands with his feet shoulder-width apart, he is more likely to turn his feet in and come up onto his toes. When they are close together, he stands better. Should I let him stand this way?"*
A. Have him stand the way he does best. But do not have him stand with legs touching. Standing with feet shoulder-width apart gives children a wider base and makes balancing easier than standing with feet close together. However, some children with cerebral palsy can control their legs better if they stand with feet close together. Aaron is one of those children.

Q. *"I am amazed that you say that doing a balance exercise with your child is like playing. When I am home from work, I enjoy hanging out with my kids on the floor. We roll around, they show me how a toy works, and similar stuff—that's playing. Tell me how a parent can hold a full-time job and have time and energy for something you're recommending?"*

A. You are right. Parents who work full time may only have time or energy for this on weekends and even then it may be very difficult for them if they have several children. You may ask for a volunteer in your church, at your neighborhood association, or within your extended family. If you find a helper to work with your child, make sure that he attends several of your child's therapy sessions so the therapist can teach him the home exercises.

Q. *"Jeff, one of the children in my early intervention preschool class, would benefit from more play in standing. However, I am concerned about his safety. I do not want him to fall and get hurt. What do you recommend?"*

A. You have a valid concern. Children with poor standing balance will fall at times. Falls cannot be 100% prevented. Talk to Jeff's parents and his physical therapist about how well Jeff is able to protect himself when falling and follow their advice. Also, when Jeff plays standing at a table, remove objects he could fall against. Children are more likely to get hurt falling against something than falling down. A carpet on the floor will provide additional protection.

15

Walking and More

"I wish Marion would walk more," her mother sighs. "It has been three months since she took her first steps and she is still reluctant to walk. I thought once children started to walk, they wanted to do it all the time. But if I don't prod Marion to walk she would rather crawl. Are there any exercises I can do with Marion to motivate her to walk?"

There are no exercises that Marion's mother needs to do with her daughter right now. Apart from continuing Marion's stretching routine, this is a good time for her parents to take a break from doing exercises with her. For Marion to walk more, faster, and for longer periods, she needs to take ownership of her new skill. Instead of walking because she is praised or prodded, she needs to walk because she wants to go somewhere or do something.

Chapter 6, *Head-Up,* talked about Nina and how important it was for her to integrate holding her head up into her daily life. In similar ways it is best for Marion's parents to stop doing walking exercises and instead help her to integrate walking into her daily routine.

Opportunities for Walking
INDOORS

All beginning walkers need time and ample opportunity to refine their new skill. Children between the ages of one and two years are called toddlers for good reasons. They totter as they learn to sort out what their legs, body, and arms have to do in order to walk faster or slower, stop and turn, step around, and move side to side or over something. It takes time and practice, and more practice for them to coordinate their movements and improve their balance.

The same is true for beginning walkers with cerebral palsy, only more so. Walking will improve with practice. Easy opportunities for walking and successful attempts will encourage them to walk more and find new challenges just right for them in their environment. At this point, parents need to become good observers, notice what their child likes, and be responsive to it.

Parents may like to plan ahead, structure their day, and be productive. It is not always convenient for them to stop what they are doing and relax, just to watch their child try something new and be ready to provide assistance if necessary. Yet, this approach is the most helpful for their child. Instead of directing their child to walk, therapists recommend that parents make the environment "walker friendly" and let the child take the initiative.

Making Walking Easy
- Open areas or hallways will help your beginning walker.
- Keep clutter at a minimum.
- Have your child or children play in one area and keep the rest of the house open for walking.
- Remove throw rugs or mats and keep your house well lighted.

Areas for Play In Standing

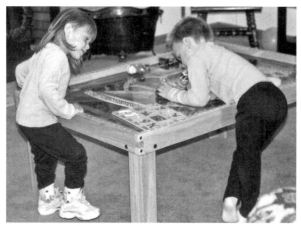

Beginning walkers like to play in standing, and the more opportunity they have for such play, the more they will walk. If they have to get down to the floor in order to play, they will most likely stay there and not practice any walking. Although they know how to stand up, it is not easy for them and crawling seems more convenient.

Here are a few ideas for play stations in standing.
- A play kitchen with a child's table placed next to it may make a good standing play area.
- A large play table with a rim will provide an ideal surface for your child with cerebral palsy and her siblings. The rim prevents building blocks, puzzle pieces, doll furnishings, or cars from falling off (photo 15.1a). And if something should drop to the floor, holding onto the rim will provide extra security for your child as he bends down to retrieve it (photo 15.1b).
  - The height of the table shown may be adjusted as your child grows (table courtesy of Nilo Toys).
- A card table placed in a corner may provide a large enough surface where a taller child may play with cars, action figures, or dolls.
- Two kitchen chairs with a wide board placed over them and strapped down with bungee cords may make a play table for a small child.
- If you have low windowsills, your child can use them as a play area.

15.1a

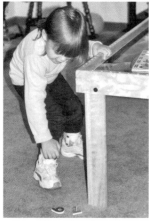

15.1b

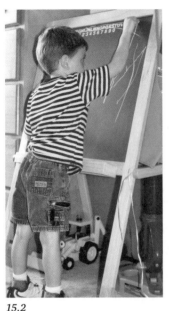

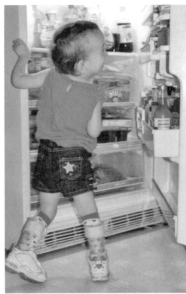

15.2　　　15.3

- An easel will provide an opportunity for your child to stand and color or finger paint (photo 15.2).
- Play with a doll carriage or a play shopping cart will encourage standing and walking.

Reasons for Standing and Walking

- Whenever your child wants a snack, have him stand up and choose something out of the refrigerator (photo 15.3). Then place it on the counter or kitchen table.
- When washing his hands or face, have him stand at the sink. When he is done, let him get the towel and use it by himself.
- Whenever you go somewhere with your child, do not carry him but have him walk with you.
- Send him to give messages to others in the family. For example: "Go tell Dad it's time to go to the library"; "Go ask Sarah what she wants to drink."

Walking and Helping

Young children love to help their parents. The beginning walker can help you by pushing something.

- Ask him to help Mom push the kitchen chairs to the table and praise him for being a good helper.
- Ask him to push the chairs away when you vacuum and later push them back in place.
- A play shopping cart is ideal for more helping tasks. Time to clean up? Have him load up his shopping cart and walk the toys back to where they belong. Time for dinner? Have him load up napkins, buns, maybe silverware into his shopping cart and push the cart to the table. Friends come to visit? With your help, he can put cans of cold soda and a bag of chips into his cart and take them to the guests.

Clutter Comes Back

When you observe that your child walks with more confidence, see if he is ready for small challenges.

- Put the throw rug or mat back in place and see if he can walk over it without tripping.
- The laundry basket sitting in the hallway may be a welcome object to walk around.

Continue to keep small things and toys out of his way, however. It may take a long time before your child is ready to step over something lying on the floor.

Carrying Objects

Have you observed your child carrying a doll, stuffed animal, or a ball? If he does so without falling or tripping you may ask him to carry things to be a good helper.

- After you have helped your child out of his coat, ask him to take it to the closet.
- Instead of having him use his shopping cart, you may ask your child to hand carry the napkins and other items to the dinner table.
- Ask him to go and get the book he wants you to read to him and to put it back on the shelf when you are done with it.
- Put his favorite videos or DVDs on top of the TV or on a shelf, so he has to stand up and walk over to the TV to get them.

Soon your child will enjoy more difficult tasks.

Opening and Closing a Door

A sliding door, like a closet door, will be easiest to open and close (photo 15.4). For safety reasons, you will have to watch your child as he tries to open or close

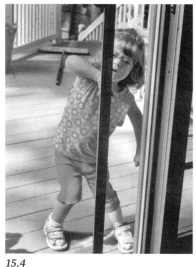

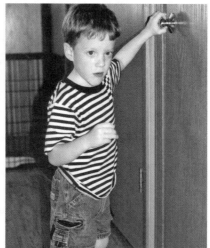

the door. This will be time consuming for you. But if your child takes the initiative and wants to do it, you may be surprised how fast he will learn. Once he is able to open the door safely on his own you may encourage him to use the skill and be a good helper by putting things in the closet.

Opening and closing a regular door may be more than he can handle at this time (photo 15.5). If you observe him trying to turn the doorknob and it proves to be too difficult for him, talk to his therapist and follow her advice.

15.4

15.5

Cleaning Up

Cleaning up a bunch of toys strewn over the floor is a big job. It means bending down, coming up, carrying the toy, and placing it where it belongs (photo 15.6). Start by asking your child to clean up two or three items and praise him for it. If he does well, have him put away more items the following week. You may be surprised how proud he will be to do this. If he has not previously been responsible for putting his own dirty clothes in the hamper, this is a good time to start.

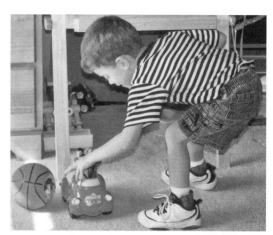

15.6

WALKING OUTDOORS AND IN PUBLIC PLACES

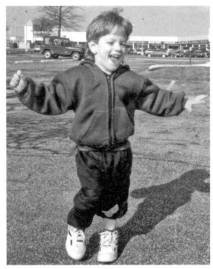

15.7

When your child walks indoors from one room to another without holding on or falling, he may also want to walk outdoors. This will bring new challenges for him. He will have to tackle wide-open spaces and will encounter rough, uneven surfaces that may be littered with debris, small sticks, stones, or leaves. His arms will be outstretched at his sides as he concentrates on walking (photo 15.7). It will not help to hold his hand because this interferes with his ability to use his arms to balance or catch himself. Holding onto his clothing will be equally counterproductive. Instead, consider the following suggestions.

Easy Walking Outside

- If you have a porch or deck, have your child venture out onto it on a dry day. Let him explore it on his own. Just watch that he doesn't try to step down from it on his own.
- If your driveway is level, he may walk there next. Park your car in the driveway and have him walk to and from it when the two of you are going somewhere or are returning. When he is not being distracted by other family members, your child will have the best chance to walk the distance successfully. As he gains confidence, he will be able to show off his new skill to the rest of the family. (Don't try this if your driveway is not level, or nearly level.)
- Park the car further away from your house and thereby increase the distance he will walk.

Walking on Grass

Your child may want to walk to your swing set, sandbox, or splashing pool. To get there, he has to walk over grass (photo 15.8). Walking on uneven surfaces such as a lawn is not easy, but it is great exercise and if he stumbles in the grass, he is less likely to hurt himself than if he falls on asphalt.

Walking and Playing

After your child has gained the confidence to walk to his preferred outside places, he will want to play there with siblings or friends.

- Playing in the sandbox will be the safest and most fun way for your beginning walker to play outside with other children.
- At the swing set, you may have a piece of equipment such as a low slide or safe swing seat that he can use and enjoy.
- Play in the driveway poses a problem for a beginning walker with cerebral palsy. The safe riding toys are often too small and the ones of the right size are often too difficult to pedal. Instead of helping him to get into or on a riding toy and pushing him around,

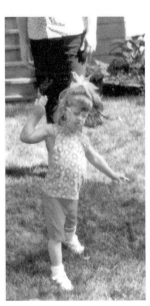

15.8

your child may have as much fun and get more exercise if you encourage him to push a toy. You may bring his shopping cart or baby carriage with his favorite doll outside for play. He may enjoy pulling a little wagon or pushing a play lawn mower.

Walking in a Mall

You may be reluctant to have your child walk into a store, the library, or any other public place. Perhaps you worry that it is too difficult for him. Carrying him or pushing him in a stroller is safer and easier. You are right in your assessment. Walking into a library or a big crowded mall is tricky for a beginning walker. Being in a busy place with all its distractions makes it harder for him to balance and concentrate on his steps.

Go to an indoor mall when there are few shoppers and see if your child is ready to walk around. If he is able to cope, have him walk as much as he likes. Provide safety by having him stay away from escalators and automatic doors that swing open. It will be great practice and exercise for him. The newness and excitement of the experience will make him walk for longer distances and teach him to focus in spite of the many distractions. It will provide valuable training for walking in school.

WALKING STAIRS

The more Marion walks, the more daring she becomes. A couple of times she tried to walk up the stairs but then decided that crawling up was still easier. When she wants to come down the stairs, she sits down and scoots down from stair to stair. During her therapy sessions, Marion practices stair walking, and as she makes progress, her therapist asks her parents to walk stairs with Marion at home.

Stair walking is an important daily living skill. Mastering it will give your child more independence. Walking up and down stairs strengthens the leg muscles and improves coordination. Stepping up, children learn to lift one leg high while standing on the other leg. Stepping down, they learn to slowly lower one leg while bringing the other leg forward to stand on it.

If your house does not have stairs, use the step up from the garage or from the front or back door into your house for practice. As there is no handrail, have your child hold onto the doorframe instead. Practice the one step step-up with your child similar to stair walking.

The following are examples of ways to practice stair walking. Use them as directed by your child's therapist and follow her specific instructions.

Walking Up Stairs Sideways

1. Ask your child to stand sideways facing the railing and hold onto it with both hands.
2. If his right side is closest to the staircase, ask him to lift his right foot up onto the first stair, lean over the right leg, push, and straighten it while lifting the left foot and placing it next to the right foot, and then stand straight.
3. Have your child move his hands up the railing and step up onto the next stair the same way and so on.

Also have your child practice this with his left leg stepping up first if your staircase has rails on both sides. Do not practice without a handrail for your child to hold onto. Good rails provide safety and make stair walking easier for your child.

Variation. If your child cannot step up or if his knee turns in:

1. As above, have your child face the rail and hold onto it. Help him step up with his right foot. The foot and knee point straight forward toward the rail.
2. Place your right hand over the right knee and stabilize it.
3. Place your left hand on his left hip and help him come up and place his left foot next to the right foot.
4. Help him in the same way to step up with his left foot first.

Walking Down Stairs Sideways

First have your child practice walking down the last few steps. Later, as he improves, he may be ready to tackle a whole flight of stairs.

1. Ask your child to stand sideways facing the railing and hold onto it with both hands.
2. Stand a step or two below and guard him well.
3. If his right side is closest to the stair, ask him to lean over his left leg, step down with his right foot by slowly bending his left leg, and place his right foot on the lower stair.
4. Then have him step down with his left leg and place the foot next to the right one.
5. Have him move his hands down the railing and step down onto the next stair in the same way and so on.
6. Next have him practice this with his left foot stepping down first.

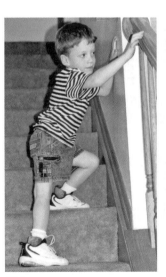 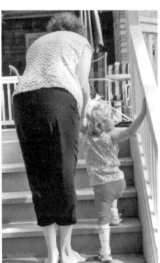

Variation. Help your child if he cannot step down or if his knee turns in:

1. Place your left hand over his left knee and your right hand on his right hip.
2. Ask or help him to point his knees and feet forward and shift his weight over his left leg.
3. Stabilize his left knee as he bends it and puts his right foot on the lower stair. Have him put his left foot down beside it without your help.
4. Help him in the same way to step down with his left leg first.

Note: When your child is able to step sideways up and down stairs safely, have him do it without any help (photo 15.9).

15.9   *15.10*

Walking Up Stairs

1. Have your child hold onto the railing with his right hand and stand with his feet pointing forward or slightly outward.
2. Hold his left hand and encourage him to walk up the stairs with you. For more assistance, you may support his upper arm with one hand and his hand with your other hand (photo 15.10)
3. Have him place first the right foot and then the left foot on each stair. Continue walking with him up the flight of stairs.
4. At a later time have him hold onto the railing with his left hand and step up with his left foot first.

Variation. Assist your child if she cannot step up or if her knees or feet turn in:
1. Have your child stand at the bottom of the stairs holding the rail with his left hand. Stand at his side and help him lift his right foot onto the step. Ask him to point the foot and knee forward.
2. You may place your right hand over his right knee and stabilize it as he brings up his left foot and places it next to the right one. With your left hand guard him from behind.
3. Next have him hold onto the railing with his right hand and walk up with his left foot first.

Note: Encourage your child to lean forward as he steps up. Do *not* have him lean backwards.

Walking Down Stairs

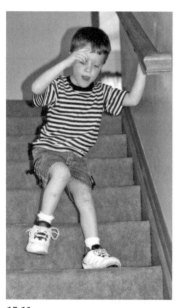

1. Have your child hold onto the railing with his left hand and stand with his feet pointing forward or slightly outward.
2. Hold his right hand and encourage him to walk down the stairs with you. Have him place first the left and then the right foot on each stair. Continue walking with him down the flight of stairs.
3. At a later time have him hold onto the railing with his right hand and step down with his right foot first.
4. Have him practice walking down on his own when he is ready for it (photo 15.11).

Variation. Assist your child if he cannot step down or if his knee turns in:
1. Instead of holding his hand, stand two or three steps below facing him. Place your left hand over his right knee. Place your right hand on his left hip or hold onto the handrail.
2. Ask and help him to stand with his feet pointing forward and to shift his weight over his right leg.
3. Stabilize his knee as he bends it and puts his left foot on the lower stair. Have him put his right foot down beside it without your help.
4. Help him in the same way when he walks down holding onto the railing with his right hand and steps down with his right leg first.

15.11

When to Practice Stair Climbing

The best time to practice is when your child needs to come up or get down the stairs for a reason. Instead of setting an extra practice time, make assisted or supervised stair walking part of your child's daily routine. If your child is independently crawling up and scooting down stairs you may be reluctant to change this. Helping him to walk down in the morning and up at night as well as other times during the day will take time. Yet the 2 to 5 minutes it will take to walk stairs with him will be time well spent. It will get him used to a stair walking routine. With constant practice he will become able to climb stairs all by himself earlier than he otherwise would.

More Advanced Stair Climbing

After your child is able to step up or down by placing both feet on each step, practice with him alternately stepping up or down by placing only one foot on each step. If you have practiced stepping up with either foot, your child may learn to walk up alternating his feet rather quickly, as long as you hold his hand. Walking down alternating feet will take more practice because it requires more coordination and balance.

Walking up stairs alternating feet with one hand on the handrail and not holding your hand will challenge your child's balance. When your child walks independently up or down the stairs, have him choose the way he feels safest. Initially, he will most likely walk up and down sideways holding onto the railing with both hands. Later, he may walk up facing forward placing both feet on each step while continuing to walk down sideways. With more practice, he may choose to alternate his feet as he walks up the stairs and come down facing forward while placing both feet on each step. Last, he will feel safe enough to walk downstairs alternating feet on his own.

Improving Balance and Coordination

Marion is walking. She walks around the house, outside, and up and down stairs. She never crawls anymore, but walks wherever she wants to go. Her parents are happy for her. At the same time, they cannot help noticing how unsteady she is. She is able to walk up the wheelchair ramp at the library but needs help walking down. She cannot step up or down a curb. At home they constantly have to remind her brother to clean up his toys. Anything in Marion's way may cause her to trip. Even stepping over a Matchbox car or train tracks is a big deal for Marion. Especially at night when she is tired, Marion easily falls. Her parents wonder how they can help Marion.

Further improvement of the coordination of their leg muscles and their balance helps children with cerebral palsy to acquire the additional skills they need for safe walking. When the children first walk, they take short steps. In order to step over an obstacle, they have to make a big step and bring their leg up high. The same is required when they want to step up a curb. To do this, the children need the muscle power to lift one leg high, the balance to temporarily bear all their weight on the other leg, and the control to slowly bend or straighten their legs.

The next activities are designed to improve your child's balance and practice controlled up and down leg movements. Use them as directed by your child's therapist and follow any specific instructions given.

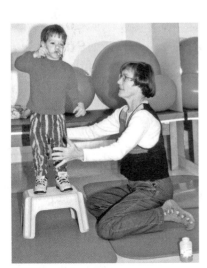

15.12

King of the Mountain

1. Place a stepping stool in a safe place in the middle of the room away from furniture or in front of your bed or your couch.
2. Have your child hold onto your hand, step up on the stool, and stand in the middle of it. His feet point straight forward or slightly turned out.
3. Encourage him to stand nice and tall, let go of your hand support, and stand on his own.
4. Count together how long he can stand all by himself. Guard him well and immediately help him to step down when he is ready or becomes unsteady.

Variation. If your child does well, let him play King of the Mountain while blowing bubbles (photo 5.12) or pretending to be an entertainer and singing for you. Continue to guard him closely while he stands on the stool.

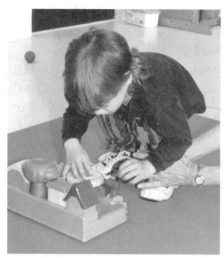

15.13a

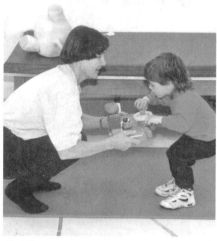

15.13b

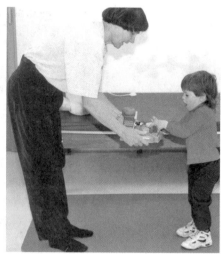

15.13c

Play in Squatting – Play in Standing

1. Place an interesting toy on the floor and have your child squat down and play with it. Make sure his feet are flat on the floor and pointing forward or slightly out (photo 15.13a).
2. After some play, slowly lift the toy (photo 15.13b) and encourage your child to slowly stand up (photo 15.13c).

Variation. Have your child squat and play with blocks, a stacking ring, a puzzle, a Color Form board, etc. Stand next to him and hold additional blocks, rings, puzzle pieces, etc. Have him stand up for a new piece and squat again for more play.

Standing on Foam

Another way to improve your child's standing balance reaction is to have him stand on a piece of dense foam. (For practice at home, you may buy a 3" thick 16 x 16" square piece of dense foam in a fabric store.)

Have your child hold onto your hands, step onto the foam square and stand with his feet pointing forward or slightly turned out.

1. Encourage him to stand nice and tall, let go of your hand support, and stand on his own (photo 15.14).
2. Together count how long he can keep his balance.
3. Have him hold onto your hands again while he steps down.

Variation. If your child does well, you may place the foam square in the middle of the room away from furniture and have him hold and bounce a ball while he stands and maintains his balance.

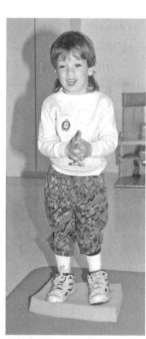

15.14

Half-Standing in front of a Mirror

Exercises in half-standing have been recommended previously for stretching the calf muscles and improving the coordination and balance of the weaker leg of a small child. They may be used for the same reasons with an older child who is already walking. Half-standing with either foot down is a good preparation for skills that require short periods of single leg standing such as stepping high, stepping up and down a curb, or climbing stairs without holding onto a railing. Use them as directed by your therapist and follow her specific instructions.

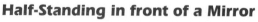

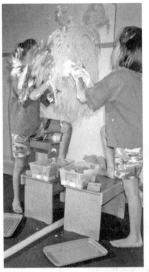

1. Place a stepstool or low bench in front of a full-length mirror or glass door. Gather the necessary supplies—shaving cream and foam blocks or foam animal shapes, as well as a towel, washcloth, and sponge for clean up.
2. Holding onto the mirror, your child places one foot on the bench with the knee and toes pointing forward. The other leg is straight at the hip and knee and the toes also point forward or slightly out.
3. Spray a blob of shaving cream on the mirror and encourage your child to spread it all around (photo 15.15). Show him how to draw a picture in the shaving cream, make handprints, or stick foam animal shapes to the mirror and then let him continue to play as long as he likes. It will be OK with you if he just messes the shaving cream all over the mirror. Protect him from falling as needed.
4. When he is done playing, have him half-stand while he cleans up with a big wet sponge. Sloshing it over the mirror will be more fun and good exercise.

15.15

Standing on One Leg

Standing on one leg is the most difficult balance skill. If children master this skill they may progress to more advanced skills such as walking on a beam, skipping, or hopping. Parents may start practicing supported one-leg standing with their children before they are walking (See Chapter 14, under the heading "Assisted Standing on One Leg").

For more one-leg standing practice, use the following exercises or activities as directed by your child's therapist.

Standing on One Leg at a Wall

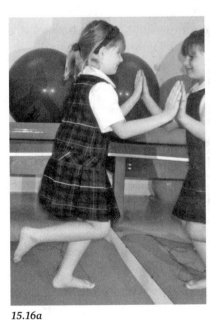

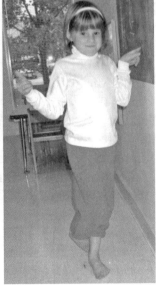

1. Your child braces himself with both hands against a wall.
2. Ask him to shift his weight onto one foot, make sure the foot points forward, and then lift the other foot (photo 15.16a). Have him:
   - Count how long he can stand on one leg.
   - Do 10 knee bends with his standing leg.
   - Come up onto toes 10 times.
3. Have him practice the same way while standing on the other leg.

Variation A. Have your child stand sideways and support himself with one hand against the wall. Have him practice standing on either leg as before.

15.16a   *15.16b*

Variation B. Have your child stand sideways and support himself with just one finger on the wall while he tries to stand on either leg for 15-30 seconds (photo 15.16b). If he is able to do this, have him exercise as before—do 10 knee bends and 10 heel rises.

Standing on One Leg

For children with cerebral palsy, the easiest way to stand on one leg is to lift the other leg out to the side. This way they can compensate for weak hip muscles. The following exercise has you practice this with your child.

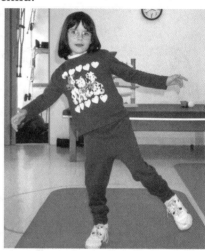

1. Your child stands with feet pointing forward or slightly outward.
2. Stand very still several feet in front of your child. Ask him to shift his weight onto one leg and lift the other leg out to the side (photo 15.17).
3. Calmly count with him how long he can balance on one leg.
4. Have him practice standing on the other leg the same way.

Variation. Practice with your child the same way, but ask him to lift his foot back and up by bending his knee.

15.17

One-Foot Beanbag Game

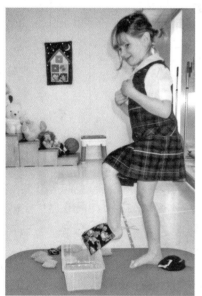

This activity makes standing on one leg fun and is a good exercise to use during playtime. It encourages concentration and good standing posture. Beanbags and a shallow box or container are needed to play it.

1. Your child stands with his back at a wall without leaning against it.
2. Place the box in front of him and put a beanbag on his foot.
3. Ask him to lift his foot and drop the beanbag into the container. If he misses, let him try again. If he succeeds, encourage him to drop another beanbag into the container, and so on, until all the bags are in the box.
4. Have him play the same way with the other foot.

Variation A. If your child does well, have him move away from the wall and let him play in the middle of the room away from any furniture he could fall on (photo 15.18).

Variation B. If your child does well and the game becomes too simple for him, challenge him by placing the box on top of a stack of books or stool, or use a taller container. Now your child has to lift his foot higher and stand longer on one leg when dropping the beanbag into the container.

15.18

The Way Your Child Walks

Marion has been walking for several years now. Her balance and endurance have improved. She no longer has to hold onto her mother's hand when she steps up onto a curb or walks down an incline. Her parents are happy for her and feel blessed. And yet, at times they observe Marion and hope she would walk even better. Instead of stepping straight forward, she swings her legs out to the side and then brings them forward. With each step, her body sways from side to side, and when she is tired her left foot turns in.

Marion's story is typical for children with cerebral palsy who walk independently. Because of the abnormal muscle tone, muscle weaknesses, and lack of coordination and balance, they walk differently than children without these problems. How much their gait differs varies from child to child. But usually there is room for improvement and parents wonder how they can help their child walk better.

Physical therapists will tell you that *the most important thing parents can do is to keep up the daily stretching routine.* Because of their walking pattern, children with cerebral palsy do not fully stretch some of their leg muscles. Without daily stretching, these muscles will shorten and the opposing muscles will become too long. Over time, this may cause your child's walking ability to decline rather than improve.

Improvement of muscle strength, coordination, and balance will help the children to walk better. Swimming, horseback riding, adapted dance, or gymnastic lessons, or any other physical fitness or sports-related activity will benefit your child. So will strengthening exercises and training programs with a stationary bike or treadmill, which the physical therapist may plan for your child. (Dodd, 03; McBurney, 03; Lowes, 04).

Another way to bring about improvement is for the therapist to train the child to walk differently. This is called gait training. It is an obvious but also a tricky solution. Walking is a continuous, repetitive movement. It not only depends on muscle strength but also on the timing and sequencing of muscle activity. Scientists are studying how people walk and still have many unanswered questions.

Most children with cerebral palsy walk as well as they are able to. Just because a child is told to step straight forward does not mean he will be able to do so. Every study done on the subject has confirmed that children with cerebral palsy use more oxygen when they walk. This means that they work harder when walking and therefore tire sooner than other children.

Physical therapists have two goals for their patients. They want them to walk with more control and to do so with less effort.

The children themselves also want to walk with as little effort as possible. When their therapist or parent asks them to change the way they walk, they feel that this new way of walking will require greater effort. Usually this is true. The walking pattern the therapist teaches will require more work and effort and will cause the child to walk slower. Only later, after practice and more practice, will the "new" way of walking become easy and energy efficient. The process of learning a new gait is very slow. Gait training is very beneficial early on when children first learn to walk, as well as later on when they are older and self-motivated.

Gait training with a very young child with cerebral palsy seems to bring minimal results. During the therapy sessions guided by the therapist, the child may walk well in parallel bars. He takes slow, controlled steps, brings his legs straight forward, and places his heels on the floor. Yet, when the session is over, he will walk out the door in the same way he walked in—using his unique pattern. His parents may wonder if the gait training is worth all the effort.

In fact, it usually *is* worth the effort. The therapist is teaching the child a new way to walk. The child is learning it by walking slowly with support. He is learning a new pattern, and, as he practices, the new way of walking becomes easier. This is valuable experience even if he is not able to integrate it in everyday life outside his therapy sessions. Later, if the child undergoes a medical intervention, which improves his muscle tone, the early training will prove very valuable. Then it will be easier for him to walk with an improved gait pattern because he will already be familiar with it and will now incorporate it into his daily life. Or, when he is about eight years or older he may decide he wants to walk "tall" and a girl may want to walk "pretty." Now the early training will help him and may make it possible, with much additional practice, for him to succeed.

The following are examples of gait training exercises. Use them as directed by your therapist and follow her specific instructions.

Walking While Straddling a Divider

This exercise is designed to train your child to step straight forward without crossing his feet in front of each other as he walks. For the exercise you need a hoop and a divider, which may be purchased from a therapy equipment supplier or constructed using a 2" x 4" board and brackets to secure the board.

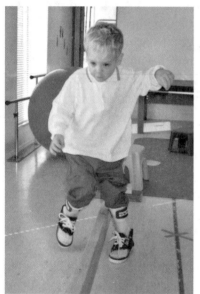
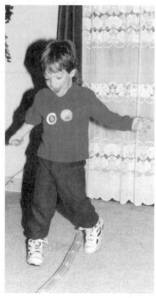

15.19a   *15.19b*

1. Place the divider on the floor. (If using a board, place it on its edge so it is 4" tall.)
2. Help your child straddle the divider at one end, with his feet flat on the floor and his toes pointing forward. Stand in front of him with a hoop for him to hold onto.
3. Ask him to slowly walk with you to the other end of the divider.
4. Assist him to turn around and walk back with you.
5. Have him walk several trips with you.

Variation A. When your child does well, encourage him to straddle the divider and walk very slowly on his own (photo 15.19a). Guard him well because you do not want him to fall onto the board. This is a very difficult exercise. Be sure to praise him after each successful trip.

Variation B. Instead of a divider, use something smaller. Place a rope, a plastic Christmas garland, or wooden train tracks on the floor. Use your imagination! Practice as before. Have your child hold onto a hoop. When he does well, have him walk without balance support (photo 15.19b).

Walking Down the Lane

This exercise is for children who walk with a wide-based gait. It challenges them to step straight forward instead of out to the side.

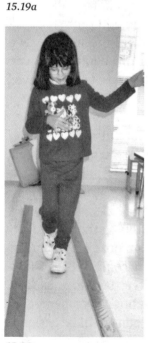

1. Set up a walkway two feet wide in a large room, on your porch or deck, or in your driveway. Mark the walkway with tape or chalk. Or use wooden slats—as used for flooring—or thick ropes to create barriers.
2. Have your child stand at one end of the walkway with his feet flat on the floor and his toes pointing forward.
3. Stand in front of your child with a hoop for him to hold onto and have him walk down the lane with you. Ask him to stay within the walkway and not step on the barriers.
4. If he does well, have him walk down the lane without support (photo 15.20). Encourage him to take many trips up and down the lane.

15.20

Variation A. When your child does well, gradually increase the length of the lane. Walking longer distances before stopping will affect the ease with which he walks and will make his gait smoother.

Variation B. When your child does well, make the lane a few inches narrower and have him practice as before—first holding onto a hoop and later without support. Begin with a short distance and gradually increase it.

Kick and Step

Marian had difficulty stepping over a toy on the floor. This is a common problem for children with cerebral palsy. To step over something, children have to balance on one leg while they lift the other leg high, straighten the knee as they kick the foot forward, and then place it on the floor. Camdon's family developed the next exercise. They first practiced with Camdon as described in Variation A. When he improved, Camdon practiced with his Dad, and Mom took the photo on the left (photo 15.21).

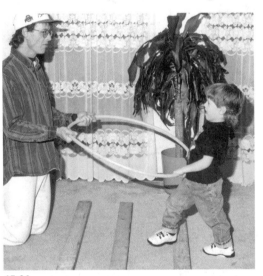

15.21

1. Place 3 to 5 wooden slats on the floor—just the right distance apart for your child to step over and between them.
2. Stand in front of him with a hoop for him to hold on to.
3. Ask him to lift and kick out his right foot and step over the first slat. Then lift and kick out the left foot and step over the next slat and so on.
4. Have him practice as long as he likes. You want your child to develop a fluid and easy stepping pattern.

Variation A. If the exercise is too difficult for your child, have him practice stepping over one slat while you hold one or both of his hands. Have him practice stepping with either leg.

Variation B. When your child is able to step over the slats with ease, have him practice without holding onto the hoop. This will challenge his balance skills and get him ready for real-life situations when he will have to step over obstacles in his path.

BRINGING FEET CLOSER TOGETHER WITHOUT TOEING IN

Walking Along a Narrow Board

The next three exercises are for children who walk with their feet far apart and with their toes turned inward. In order to do the exercises, the children may have to walk very slowly and concentrate on each step. Holding onto a hoop will help them initially. Use the exercises as directed by your child's therapist and follow any specific instructions.

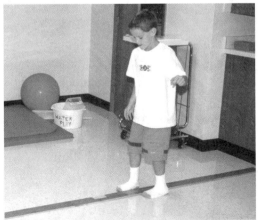

15.22

1. Place several wooden slats in a row on the floor and have your child straddle them so that his heels are very close to the edges and his feet are pointing forward.
2. Ask him to walk very slowly, always placing his heels close to the barrier without stepping on it with his forefeet (photo 15.22). If needed, have him walk with you, holding onto a hoop or onto sticks. If he loses control and places his heel away from the slat, ask him to stop, place his feet into the starting position and then begin to walk again.

Sliding Along

When wearing thick white socks, your child can practice the following exercise on a smooth and slippery floor.

1. Have your child stand with his feet straight forward.
2. With a marker draw a forward-pointing arrow on each sock. These arrows will give him a visual cue that will help him keep his feet pointing straight ahead.
3. Now ask him to keep the feet on the floor and alternately slide them forward as if he were skating.

Walking Straight Forward

1. On a piece of cardboard or poster board, draw two arrows about 1.5" inches wide and 4 to 7" inches long. Cut out the arrows and tape them onto the tops of your child's shoes so that the arrows point straight forward. The arrows should extend less than an inch beyond the shoes. Otherwise they may cause your child to trip and fall.
2. Ask him to walk so the arrows will always point forward (photo 15.23). If necessary, ask him to walk very slowly with you and hold onto a hoop or two sticks you hold.

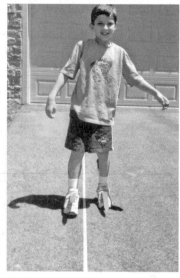

15.23

WEIGHT BEARING OVER THE HEELS

When children with cerebral palsy stand, they may have most of their weight shifted over their forefeet instead of equally distributed over their forefeet and heels. Learning to stand and balance with 50 percent or more of their weight over their heels will be beneficial for these children. It increases the size of their base of support. This will also improve their standing balance in the backward direction—for instance, if they are pushed backwards, they will be able to use their heels to help maintain their balance and prevent a fall. It will make it easier for them to step backwards and it may also help them to put their heels down first as they are walking forward.

The next exercises train weight bearing over the heels. Use them as directed by your child's therapist.

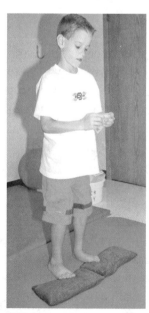

Standing with Toes Up

- Your child stands with his back against a wall and his toes and forefeet placed on a sandbag, beanbag, or ¾" thick strip of foam block. (For a small child, use only a ½" thickness of foam block.) Now more of your child's weight is over his heels.
- Ask him not to lean forward but to relax, stand straight, and lean against the wall if necessary.
- Have him stand this way for 3–5 minutes while quietly playing with a handheld toy.
- When your child's balance has improved, have him practice standing away from the wall (photo 15.24).

15.24

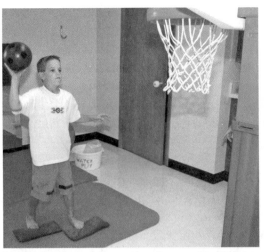

15.25

Step Forward Standing with Toes Up

1. Your child stands sideways next to a wall—ready to support himself with one hand as needed. Ask him to stand with one foot a step ahead of the other, with knees apart and toes pointing forward.
2. Place a sandbag, beanbag, or ½" piece of foam block under his toes and forefeet.
3. Encourage him to relax, balance without holding onto the wall, and quietly play with a handheld toy for 3 to 5 minutes.
4. Whenever your child is ready, have him practice standing like this away from the wall while doing an activity such as shooting baskets (photo 15.25). Have him practice with either foot forward.

Frequently Asked Questions

Q. *"We believe that gait training exercises may help our daughter Myla. Should we do all of them with her?"*

A. No. Talk to Myla's physical therapist. He will tell you which ones are right for Myla. Most likely he will practice them with Myla and then show you how to do them at home.

Q. *"Should we do the exercises with Myla every day?"*

A. Yes, daily practice is best. If this is not possible, do them several times a week.

Q. *"How long should Myla practice the exercises?"*

A. Keep the exercise routine up as long as Myla is making progress. Look for the small signs of weekly progress. Initially, Myla may need to hold onto a hoop, walk very slowly, and have to stop and fix her feet after a few steps. After a week or two, she may only hold onto your finger. Next, she may be able to do more good steps in a row, and so on.

Q. *"If we practice for 10 days and Myla makes no progress with the exercises, should we stop practicing?"*

A. No, as a general rule I recommend that you use a new exercise for three weeks before you make a decision like that. In addition, it will always be best if you share any concern about the exercises as soon as possible with Myla's therapist.

Q. *"Oliver is 8 years old. He has been walking since age 3, but he still does not like to walk in a store. Why do you recommend that parents take their child to a mall? I would never do this."*

A. All children are different. Since Oliver does not like to be in a store, you made the right decision by not taking him there. Nevertheless, that does not mean that another child could not benefit from walking in a mall.

Q. *"Our daughter Karen is in second grade. Her teacher wants me to bring Karen's wheelchair to school on library day because it would be too far for Karen to walk to the library. I know the distance and I know Karen can handle it. What should I do?"*
A. Talk to Karen's teacher and find out more about her request. Maybe she feels Karen would get too tired from walking or it would take her too long. Also talk to the school physical therapist and to Karen. Why not let Karen walk to the library a few times, see how it works out, and then make a decision? This is the course of action I would recommend.

Q. *"Tom is 10 years old. When he was small he needed braces to keep him from toe walking. Lately he has started to walk with bent knees and we have been taking him to physical therapy again. Why did this happen and will therapy help?"*
A. Children with cerebral palsy frequently start to walk with bent knees at Tom's age. It is called a crouch or sinking gait. Therapy combined with spasticity management will help Tom. There are several things you can do:

1. Help Tom do daily leg stretches. This will assure that Tom does not lose the flexibility of his hamstring muscles and the ability to straighten the knee.
2. If Tom is able to stand straight, remind him to do so routinely. Walking with bent knees puts stress on the knee joint. So you want to make sure that he relieves the stress and straightens his knees when he stands. Another way to reduce stress to the knee would be for Tom to use forearm crutches whenever he has to walk longer distances.
3. Have Tom do 15 to 20 minutes of leg strengthening exercises 3 to 4 times a week. Tom's therapist will be the best person to give you an exercise program. The exercises Lift Off, Wall Slides, and Heel Rises, listed in the next chapter under the heading Extra Strengthening Exercises, could be part of Tom's exercise program.

Q. *"Rose is 5 years old and walking on her own. But she is unsteady. We plan a family vacation at the beach. I worry that walking on the beach will be too difficult for Rose. What do you think?"*
A. Walking in the soft sand will be more difficult for Rose than walking on a hard surface. She may want to hold onto your hands. At the same time, it will be very good for her feet. Walking barefoot in the sand will exercise and stretch her foot muscles. Rose may have a great time playing in the sand. I would not be surprised if Rose will enjoy the beach vacation very much.

Common sense safety measures should be followed. For instance, have Rose wear a lifejacket and make sure a parent is close by when she plays near the surf.

Q. *"Our house sits on an elevation. When our children play outside, they have to walk up and down our lawn or driveway. Our daughter, Iris, was just diagnosed with cerebral palsy. We wonder if we should move to a house on level ground?"*
A. Wait and see how Iris will develop. It may turn out that walking up and down your driveway or lawn will be very good exercise for her. If not, you could always move at a later time.

16

Extra Strengthening and Having Fun

Strengthening Exercises

Strong muscles work better than weak muscles. Good muscle strength will help your child to sit or stand taller, walk better, and improve her endurance and stamina. Being physically fit helps all people, including children with cerebral palsy or similar movement disorders.

So far, the focus of this book has been on teaching new motor skills. After years of learning, there will come a time when your child has reached her potential. She may do well with her transfer skills. She may walk safely. She may walk stairs and negotiate curbs without help. "Is there still a need for more exercises?" you wonder. Yes, there is. Exercises will help your child maintain her skills as she grows older and her body changes.

For many children with cerebral palsy, transfer skills or walking may never become easy automatic skills, but always require some extra attention and effort. A typically developing child may learn a motor skill such as ice skating, walking on stilts, or riding a unicycle. However, if she does not remain physically fit and agile, she may no longer do the skill well or even lose it. Likewise, a child with cerebral palsy may no longer walk as well as previously if her lifestyle, body weight, or size changes, or her fitness level deteriorates due to an illness or a surgery.

Daily stretches and a set of exercises are the best way for the children to stay fit and maintain their independence throughout childhood, adolescence, and adulthood.

The following are four popular strength exercises. Each exercise strengthens a different muscle group. The exercises were chosen because they can easily be adapted

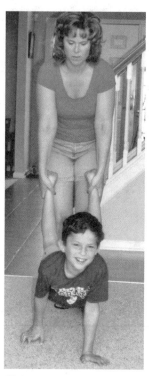

16.1

to a specific child's level of ability. They may be used to build up your child's level of strength or to maintain it. They may become part of a daily workout session. Your child's physical therapist will give you specific numbers of repetitions or goals for each exercise and combine them with other exercises your child may benefit from. Use them as directed by the therapist and follow her specific instructions.

Wheelbarrow Walking

This exercise strengthens the shoulder and arm muscles. Arm and shoulder strength is important for children with cerebral palsy. They allow the child who uses an assistive device to walk with more ease. For a child in a wheelchair, it makes transfers easier. For a walking child, strong arms provide safety during a fall.

1. Support your child's thighs, knees, or ankles while she walks on her hands (photo 16.1). The lower down on her legs you support her, the more strenuous is the exercise.
2. Have your child do this as far or for as many minutes as directed by your physical therapist.

Lift Off

This exercise strengthens your child's back muscles. Children with cerebral palsy usually have weak back muscles and benefit from this exercise very much. This is true for children who use a wheelchair as well as for children who walk independently.

1. Support your child as she lies on her stomach on a bed, bench, etc. with her head and shoulders extending over the edge, as shown in photo 16.2.
2. Ask her to "lift off" by raising herself up like an airplane. Firmly hold her bottom down while she straightens her trunk and stretches out her arms.

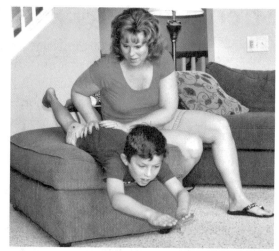

16.2

3. Encourage her to fly straight, curve to either side, tip her wings, etc.
4. Have her play as long as directed by your physical therapist.

The longer she flies, the more strenuous is the exercise. The exercise is easier if only the upper part of the chest is unsupported and harder if most of the trunk is suspended over the edge of the furniture.

Wall Slides

This is a leg muscle strengthening exercise. It strengthens specifically the quadriceps, especially so if done with one leg at a time. Good quadriceps strength prevents or reduces crouching. Have your child do this exercise for as many repetitions and as frequently per week as her therapist advises.

1. Your child stands with her back against a wall. Her feet are shoulder-width apart and her toes point forward or slightly outward (photo 16.3a).

2. Ask her to bend her knees and slowly slide as far downward as possible without lifting the heels off the floor (photo 16.3b).
3. Then have her slowly come up until her knees and hips are completely straight.
4. Repeat as often as directed by your physical therapist

Asking your child to lift one leg off the floor and then do the knee bends with the other leg will make the exercise more strenuous.

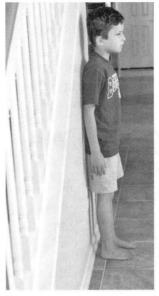
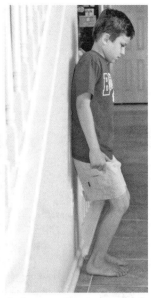

16.3a   *16.3b*

Heel Rises

This is a calf muscle strengthening and stretching exercise. Calf muscles are important for good standing balance. During walking they provide push off for efficient walking. Have your child do this exercise as frequently per week as her therapist advises.

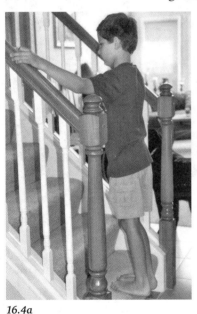

1. Your child stands on the first stair step holding onto the banisters with both hands.
2. Help her to stand on her forefeet (roughly from the toes to the instep) with the heels unsupported (photo 16.4a).
3. Ask her to slowly lift herself up on toes (photo 16.4b) and then slowly lower her heels as far as possible.
4. Repeat as often as directed by your physical therapist.
5. Good arm support makes the exercise easier. Lightly touching the banister makes it harder.
6. Lifting one leg and practicing single leg heel raises will make the exercise more strenuous.

16.4a   *16.4b*

Having Fun

Children with cerebral palsy benefit from outdoor or indoor physical activities as much or even more than other children do. But due to their physical limitations, they tend to spend more time indoor and more time sitting. This is a concern for parents who like an active, healthy lifestyle for their children. The following are examples of activities that parents have reported their child with cerebral palsy enjoyed. The first activities are for young children and the last ones are for older children.

Moving along on a Riding Toy

One mother tells us: "I place my hands over my son's hands on the handlebars and we race around the house. It's a lot of fun. He stays on the riding toy and is learning to hold on by himself (photo 16.5a)."

The child in photo 16.5b shows that he can sit and hold on without help. Next he will try to push forward.

Pushing off with their feet and riding forward is not easy for children with cerebral palsy. First, practice with your child getting on and off the riding toy—with your assistance as needed. Once he can do both safely, you may encourage him to pedal on his own. If your child cannot get off on his own, he still may enjoy sitting on the toy and move about with your help. But do not have him sit on the toy unattended.

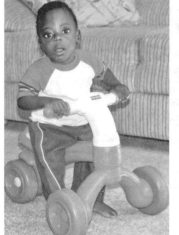

16.5a

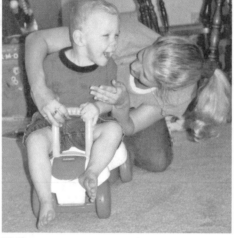

16.5b

My Rocking Horse

The boy in photo 16.6 loves his rocking horse. He rides it in the kitchen and watches Mom as she gets dinner ready.

If you have a small rocking horse for your child, teach her to hold on well with both hands. Gently rock her while you support her as needed. After she sits well on her own and consistently holds on with both hands, you may have her rock on her own.

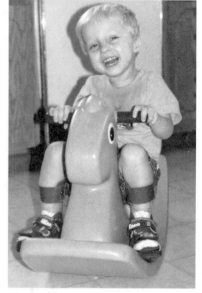

16.6

A Swing for Me

Sitting in a swing is a treat for the girl in photo 16.7. Dad mounted one for her in the playroom. Now she can enjoy it even on a rainy day. Pushing her is a relaxing and bonding time for mother and daughter.

Pushing a Toy

Push toys are easy for a child with poor balance to use. There are a great variety of them available. Parents report that their children like to take them outside as they join other children in play.

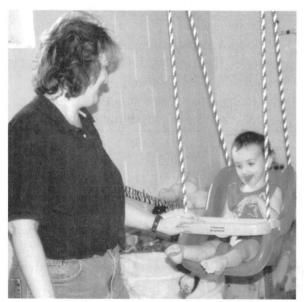

16.7

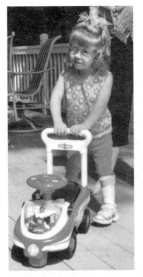
16.8a

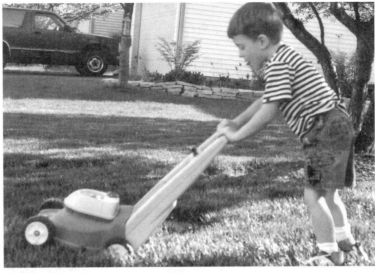
16.8b

Holding on with both hands, the girl in photo 16.8a enjoys pushing a toy along the deck. The boy in photo 16.8b pretends to mow the lawn.

Riding a Battery-Powered Riding-On Toy

The boy in photo 16.9 enjoys riding his Power Wheels. These types of battery-powered riding toys do not provide the exercise of a tricycle or bicycle. But they allow the child who cannot ride a trike or bike to join his friends outside. For a child who may use an electric wheelchair at a later time, a battery-powered vehicle means freedom of movement and valuable training in steering and maneuvering.

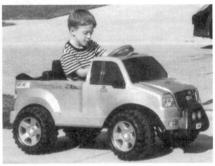
16.9

Pedaling a Tricycle

Riding a tricycle trains balance and coordination and strengthens the leg muscles. But most of all it is fun. The child in photo 16.10a has difficulty walking but enjoys riding his adapted tricycle.

One father mounted the cut-off seat of a baby swing onto his daughter's tricycle. Now she sits safely on her tricycle while she is learning to pedal (photo 16.10b).

If you want your child to ride a tricycle, ask your physical therapist for advice or assistance. Most early intervention or outpatient

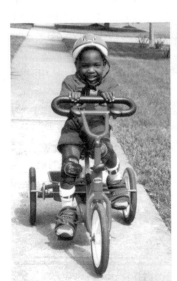
16.10a

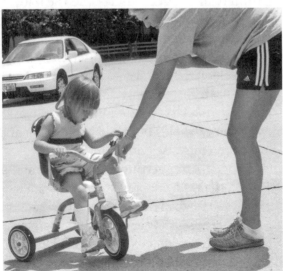
16.10b

programs have a variety of tricycles for your child to practice on and to find the most suitable trike for your child.

In general, children with cerebral palsy are significantly older than other children before they become able to ride a tricycle. For your small child just to sit, to hold onto the handlebar, and to steer is a big accomplishment. She may enjoy doing this while you push her around. A tricycle with a push handle will make this easy for you.

Some children with cerebral palsy or other movement disorders do not like to ride a tricycle even though their parents and physical therapists believe that they should be able to do it and would have fun if they did. If your child is one of those children, remember that tricycle riding is not an essential motor skill.

Playing Ball

T-ball, softball, baseball, basketball, volleyball, bowling, miniature golf, golf, and soccer are sports that youngsters with cerebral palsy or similar movement disorders

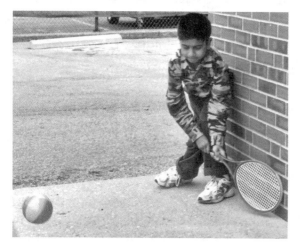

may enjoy in modified form or even in their regular forms. If your child is able to stand and walk without arm support, it may not be too difficult to find a ball activity she may enjoy playing with you or her siblings in your yard. She may even like to play on a team with typically developing children. Finding an opportunity for a child who uses a walking aid is more difficult. Top Soccer is a program, which helps children enjoy soccer in spite of their limitations. If your child is interested in soccer, find out if your community has such a program.

At home parents may find creative ways for their child to play ball. The youngster in photo 16.11 walks with a forward walker. Asked about his favorite activity, he answered, "Playing cricket." Leaning against the wall he is safe, can concentrate on the ball his father throws, and bats it right back.

16.11

Swimming

Swimming, especially in warm water, is very beneficial to children with cerebral palsy. The warmth relaxes tight muscles and the buoyancy of the water encourages

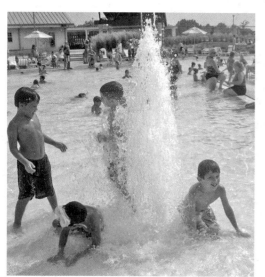

movements. Splashing with their arms, children have fun and strengthen their arm, shoulder, and back muscles. Kicking with their legs, they strengthen their hip and leg muscles. Even babies enjoy the water and benefit from it. Find out if your community has a heated pool that offers parent/infant swim classes or adapted swim classes. Attending such a class with your child teaches you how to hold your child in the water and about safe flotation devices you may use with her.

After getting used to the water and liking it, your child may attend an adapted swim program at a later time. It will teach her to be safe in the water and to swim. Swimming is a wonderful lifetime sport for a person with cerebral palsy. Before your child has acquired water safety skills, she will need your direct supervision even in shallow water. This does not mean that your child cannot have plenty of fun by the water. The youngster in photo 16.12a

16.12a

enjoys hanging out at the fountain by the pool. At the beach he proudly shows off the sandcastle he has built (photo 16.12b).

Note: Aquatic Therapy is a physical therapy method, which teaches exercises in water. Its goal is to achieve specific treatment objectives. Aquatic therapists do not teach swimming.

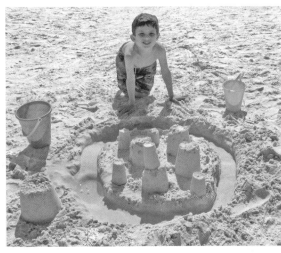

16.12b

Horseback Riding

Horseback riding is the favorite sport of many children with cerebral palsy. Besides being fun, it improves the children's posture, balance, and range of motion. It provides them with an enriching experience which gives them confidence and boosts their self-esteem. If you believe that your child may enjoy horseback riding, find out if your community has a therapeutic riding program for children with special needs. Such a program would provide the safest way to introduce your child to riding. If your child learns to ride independently, he may join other children in regular riding classes later. Potentially, horse back riding may develop into a lifetime sport.

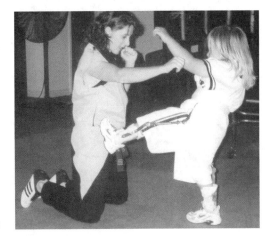

16.13

The youngster in photo 16.13 started to ride his horse, Buddy, when he was five. Now a teenager, he treasures his time with Buddy.

Note: Hippotherapy differs from therapeutic riding. It is a treatment method that uses the horse and its movements to reach specific treatment goals. The person conducting hippotherapy has to be a certified instructor of this treatment method.

Martial Arts

Karate, Kung-Fu, and Tae kwon do improve your child's standing posture and balance. As she learns to do quick kicks, controlled falls, and turns, she gains better motor control. In addition, the sports pride themselves in promoting confidence and self-respect by teaching self-discipline, concentration, respect, and courtesy. Martial arts are not team sports. Therefore, they may be adapted to an individual child's level of competence.

16.14

If you think that you child would have fun doing this type of sport, check whether your community has a special program or a teacher qualified to work with your child. The child in photo 16.14 on the previous page attends a Tae kwon do class and receives some individual instructions. Even though she still uses a walker for longer trips, she enjoys the training very much and loves to show off to her physical therapist each new trick she has learned.

Dance Lessons

Dance improves your child's posture, balance, and motor control. Group lessons encourage turn taking, attention, cooperation, and discipline. It will booster your child's self-esteem and confidence. But most of all, moving with music is fun. Getting dressed up and showing off new skills may be more fun for an outgoing child. If your community has an adapted dance class for children with special needs, you may check it out and see if you child likes it. Children with milder forms of cerebral palsy (Level I of the Gross Motor Function Classification System) may enjoy regular dance classes.

17

Additional Interventions for Children with Cerebral Palsy By Lisa Barnett, DPT

The previous chapters in this book explore many of the concepts and activities crucial to optimizing gross motor development in children with cerebral palsy and similar movement disorders. Many of these involve activities and exercises that parents can do with their child at home with the guidance of a physical therapist. However, there are other interventions that are vital to helping children with cerebral palsy achieve the best possible gross motor function. These include medical procedures such as surgery or medication, as well as bracing and serial casting. This chapter will attempt to give you some key information about these other interventions that your physical therapist might suggest to help improve the function of your child.

The goal of this chapter is not to present every piece of evidence about a procedure or to advocate which treatment or type of equipment you should use for your child. Each child and family has their unique story and needs. The goal of this chapter is instead to introduce you to a number of important topics to better educate you before you set out on your own medical journey with your child. Reading this chapter should give you increased knowledge and confidence as you consult with professionals involved with your child to gain more information on each of these and other treatment options.

Medical Management

There is no medical treatment that can cure a child of his cerebral palsy. Medications and surgery can, however, reduce spasticity, improve muscle length, and reduce joint limitations, which can, in turn, make it easier for these children to achieve gross motor skills.

The types of medical treatment I will briefly review in this chapter are:
- medications taken by mouth to reduce muscle tone,
- the intrathecal baclofen pump (IBP),
- botulinum toxin injections (Botox), and
- selective dorsal rhizotomy (SDR).

I will also discuss several interventions that may be suggested by your physical therapist. These include serial casting, neuromuscular stimulation, and lower extremity (leg) bracing.

ORAL MEDICATIONS

Some of the more common medications used to help decrease muscle tone in children with cerebral palsy include baclofen, dantrium, zanaflex, and valium. All of these drugs are oral medications, which mean they are taken by mouth, travel through the gastrointestinal tract, and then enter the bloodstream. Often these oral medications are prescribed before any more invasive medical intervention is considered, although this is not always the case. One of the drawbacks with oral medications is that they have an effect on the entire body, and thus are not as specific to the spastic muscles as other medical interventions that will be discussed.

Before any medication is started, it is important to establish goals for the use of the medication with the professionals caring for your child. If the medication is effective for your child, improvements might be seen in increased range of motion, better tolerance to braces, a gain in functional skills, or easier management by the family during daily care activities. It is equally important to make specific plans to evaluate the effect of the medication after a certain period of time to determine if the goals have been met. This will help you and your professional team decide whether your child should continue to take the medication and whether the current dosage is correct.

As with all medications, there is always the possibility of unwanted side effects. Drowsiness is one of the more common side effects of medications to reduce muscle tone. Consult with your child's physician to learn more about both the positive and negative effects that you might observe with a specific medication.

INTRATHECAL BACLOFEN

Baclofen is presently the drug most often used in the treatment of children with cerebral palsy who have moderately or severely increased muscle tone. Baclofen can be given either by mouth or through a small pump that is surgically placed in the abdomen. The pump delivers the medication to the spinal cord through a small tube, which is threaded under the skin to the spinal cord. Baclofen administered through the pump is called intrathecal baclofen (ITB).

Children considered for the pump typically have high muscle tone that involves the arm, leg, and trunk muscles and that either interferes with their daily care activities or causes them discomfort. For example, a parent might report difficulty diapering or bathing their child as a result of the high muscle tone.

Children with joints that cannot be moved through the full range of motion are not usually candidates, as the baclofen will not correct these joint contractures. Coupled with daily stretching, however, baclofen may help prevent future joint contractures by reducing the high muscle tone.

When a child has a pump surgically implanted, family members take on a serious commitment and high level of responsibility. Implantation of the pump requires a hospital admission of two to six days. The pump must be refilled in a qualified physician's office every one to three months depending on the size of the pump. If the medication is stopped or significantly reduced over a short period of time, baclofen withdrawal can quickly become an emergency situation. This is why consistent medical supervision and routine follow-up care are so important.

BOTULINUM TOXIN

Botulinum toxin (Botox) is just one of many different types of injections that are given to reduce spasticity. Alcohol, phenol, and Bupivicaine are also types of injections that are given to reduce spasticity, but these are not as commonly used for children with cerebral palsy. I will focus here on botulinum toxin and its use for reduction of spasticity in children with cerebral palsy.

There are seven types of botulinum toxin, labeled A through G. Type A, often called Botox, is the most common type and is now used in its purified form as a medicine to reduce muscle spasticity, as well as cosmetically to reduce wrinkles. Botulinum toxin is derived from Clostridum Botulinum, a gram positive bacteria frequently associated with contaminated food. In its unpurified form, this toxin is the cause of human botulism. The purified medicinal form of Botulinum toxin will be our focus.

The purified form of botulinum toxin is an especially effective medicine because of its specific action at the junction of the nerve and muscle. One therapeutic principle behind the use of botulinum toxin is that the spasticity present in some muscles in children with cerebral palsy covers up underlying muscle weakness of other closely associated muscles. With the use of botulinum toxin, the idea is to temporarily wipe out this overlying spasticity by injecting the liquid toxin directly into a spastic muscle. Then all of the child's muscles can be more aggressively strengthened and stretched during the three- to six-month time the botulinum toxin is effective. Following botulinum toxin injections, the frequency of physical therapy is usually increased in order to maximize the results gained by this intervention.

The advantages of botulinum toxin injections are:
- they cause little pain,
- they can be given in a clinic setting,
- there is an easy and rapid delivery of medicine to the desired muscle sites,
- the effects are reversible, and
- the injections can be repeated in the future if required.

The botulinum toxin injection buys the child with spastic muscles some time, which may allow his muscle growth/length to catch up with his bone growth. This, in turn, may postpone or prevent the need for orthopedic surgery.

Children with many types of cerebral palsy with varying levels of spasticity can be appropriate candidates for these injections. In general, these injections are used to target specific muscles that are interfering with your child's function. The most common sites for botulinum toxin use in the legs are the inner thigh muscles (adductors), the muscles in the back of the thigh (hamstrings), and the calf muscle (gastrocnemius). Less commonly, botulinum toxin injections may also be used for spastic muscles in the arm and hand. Consult with your therapist and physician to help you determine if your child should be considered for this treatment.

SELECTIVE DORSAL RHIZOTOMY

Selective dorsal rhizotomy (SDR) is an irreversible neurosurgical procedure for children with spastic cerebral palsy. This type of surgery is usually done only in large regional centers that see a great number of children with cerebral palsy. The operation involves surgery on the spinal cord, specifically selected dorsal roots of the spinal cord that are sending abnormal information from the muscles to the brain.

There are two different types of nerve roots in the spinal cord that transmit information to and from the muscles and the brain. The ventral (motor) spinal roots send information from the brain to the muscles. The dorsal (sensory) roots send information that is sensed by the muscles to the brain. It is these dorsal roots that a selective dorsal rhizotomy targets because some of these roots, made up of rootlets, send abnormal and distorted information to the brain, which results in spastic muscles. Only the most abnormal roots are cut, resulting in a reduction of abnormal messages and thus removing some of the spasticity.

With less spasticity, children have more control over their movement patterns and are then able to better improve their strength and balance skills. This surgery usually targets the legs, including the muscles of the hip, and typically results in improved walking for your child. As with any surgery, there are risks involved and these should be discussed extensively prior to surgery.

Candidates for selective dorsal rhizotomy usually have spastic diplegia, are between the ages of two and ten, have good underlying muscle strength, have the potential to progress to walking, and are within the average range of intelligence. Cognitive abilities are a consideration because recovery after this surgery will require extensive rehabilitation to maximize the surgical outcome. In some instances, this surgery may also be recommended for children with severe spastic quadriplegia with intelligence below the average range. The goals of surgery for these more severely involved children are related to the child's comfort, ease of care, and quality of life.

It is important to remember that spasticity is not the only symptom seen in children with cerebral palsy. This surgery cannot directly correct poor balance, muscle weakness, and abnormal movement patterns. The surgery will remove some of the spasticity, which is the underlying cause of limited range of motion, but it will not correct a permanently shortened muscle or joint contracture. In some cases, orthopedic surgery will be necessary to correct these fixed limitations.

If your physician and physical therapist believe your child might be a candidate for selective dorsal rhizotomy, you and your child will likely be referred to a regional center for assessment by a team of professionals who specialize in this type of surgery and rehabilitation. The rehabilitation after a selective dorsal rhizotomy is intensive; it can last six months to one year, and requires significant support and commitment of the family. Your child will need physical therapy three to five times a week for the first six months. You will be expected to assist your child in completing exercises at home on a daily basis to ensure the best possible outcome.

Serial Casting

Even though parents may faithfully stretch their child's muscles, it is sometimes not possible to prevent limitations in range of motion. When this occurs, discussion with your therapist or physician may result in a recommendation for serial casting. This intervention is often used prior to consideration of any orthopedic surgery. Serial casting consists of a series of casts that are applied to increase the length of specific muscles, most often at the ankles, but occasionally also for the knees or elbows. Serial casting is most often completed in a hospital or outpatient clinic by a physical therapist who specializes in casting.

If your child has the ability to walk, the casts will be designed so that he or she will be able to continue to walk with the casts in place. The casts are applied with the joints in a stretched out position and are usually left in place for five to seven days to allow the muscles to adjust to the new lengthened position.

A second set of new casts is then applied which should reflect the newly gained range of motion from the first set. This will be repeated for several weeks until the desired range of movement has been gained. Thus, the name serial casting refers to a series of casts that your child will wear, each one reflecting the gained range of motion from the previous one.

After your child's range of motion is increased and the final set of casts is removed, a program will be planned to help maintain this increased range of motion. In addition to resuming the daily stretching activities, specific exercises and night splinting may be recommended. It is not unusual for children with cerebral palsy to have serial casts applied every one to two years, especially during periods of rapid growth.

Neuromuscular Electrical Stimulation

Neuromuscular electrical stimulation (NMES) is a treatment option that is used to help children who have cerebral palsy learn which muscles should be working during a functional activity such as walking. It is used to increase sensory awareness and further stimulate and strengthen the muscles the child is using or should be using during the selected functional activity. Although there are other types and uses of electrical stimulation, this chapter focuses on NMES because of its well documented use for children with cerebral palsy.

Neuromuscular electrical stimulation is the application of electrical current to muscles to help them contract. The electrical signal is transmitted by a small, battery-operated electrical stimulation machine usually held by the physical therapist. The electrical signal travels between two electrodes, similar to small pads, that are placed on the child's skin, and the signal is transmitted to the specific muscle. This stimulation initially feels like a small tingly sensation. As the child acclimates to the stimulation, the intensity is gradually increased to a therapeutic threshold level that is tolerable to him.

Neuromuscular electrical stimulation is only successful when children are active participants in this treatment and they are encouraged to anticipate and initiate movement. Active participation is necessary for motor learning to occur. One important desired outcome with this treatment is the carry over of the appropriate movement into the child's life without the use of neuromuscular electrical stimulation. This treatment would therefore not be appropriate for a child without motor learning ability. Neuromuscular electrical stimulation is usually used in a physical therapy clinic or office, although it can become part of a home program if you and your therapist determine that this is effective. Consult with your therapist for further information related to this intervention.

Lower Extremity Bracing

Braces (orthoses) are devices made out of strong, flexible plastic that are used to improve gross motor function in children and adults with orthopedic disorders. They are worn on the lower extremities, usually at the ankles. Most children with cerebral palsy wear lower extremity braces at some point in their lives to assist them with more independent functioning. In this section, I will focus on common bracing concepts for the lower extremities.

Children with cerebral palsy have braces prescribed for a variety of problems. One common reason for wearing braces is to maintain range of motion and so prevent joint contractures that develop when muscles with increased tone remain in a shortened position over long periods of time. The brace will keep the specific muscle or muscles in a lengthened state, which allows your child the best possible function and may prevent the need for orthopedic surgery in the future.

Braces may also be suggested to help improve your child's walking pattern. Children who walk on their toes or with knees bent due to spastic, overactive calf muscles and/or weak thigh muscles may be able to get their heels down and/or knees straight when provided with bracing to control the unwanted movements caused by the spastic muscles. Children with weakness underlying the spastic calf muscles may show poor heel-to-toe foot placement or frequent stubbing of the toes while walking. Braces that support these weak muscles usually result in an improved walking pattern.

Children with poor foot alignment in standing, such as those with flattened arches and/or clenched toes, frequently show improved standing alignment and posture when their foot position is corrected and supported by bracing. These are just a few of the common problems that respond to bracing. It is important to remember that each child has his own unique bracing needs that will require equally unique problem solving to meet these needs.

TYPES OF BRACES

In deciding what kind of bracing would best help your child, you and your child's physical therapist should consider two key building blocks. You should consider the position that allows your child maximum function of the body part that is to be braced, and you should consider how much control is needed to achieve this maximum function. For example, if your child needs bracing at the foot and ankle, the first question to ask is, "What is the position of greatest function for his foot and ankle"? The second question to ask is, "How much control of the foot and ankle do we need to use to effectively brace him? Specifically, what movements do we restrict and what do we allow to move freely to get and keep the foot in the position of greatest function? These two key elements drive the decision-making process in choosing which type of bracing will work best for an individual child.

Below are descriptions of the types of braces commonly used for children with cerebral palsy. These are typically used to better align the foot, ankle, and lower leg for improved posture and function, and to assist the child in stance and walking.

Ankle Foot Orthoses (AFOs). One of the most frequently prescribed type of brace is the ankle foot orthosis (commonly called AFO), which is used to control the ankle and foot. An AFO wraps around the foot and ankle and fits inside the child's shoe. The usual purpose of the AFO is to better align the foot and restrict unwanted ankle movement so your child does not walk on his toes. AFOs can either be rigid or hinged at the ankle, depending on the child's need. AFOs are usually used for children with increased tone in their legs to help increase their stability and so improve their standing and walking.

Dynamic Ankle Foot Orthoses (DAFOs). For children with abnormal muscle tone who are more active, dynamic ankle foot orthoses, or DAFOs, may be recommended. The DAFO is made of a thinner, more flexible plastic that provides the minimum support and control needed by your child, thus allowing him to use his own abilities when possible. The DAFO usually wraps around the whole foot, accentuates the arches of the foot, and raises the toes with the goal of decreasing increased tone in the feet.

Supramalleolar Orthoses (SMO). For children who are able to control ankle movement but need more precise foot control, supramalleolar orthoses, or SMOs, may be prescribed. The SMO wraps around the foot but only comes slightly above the child's ankle. Supramalleolar refers to above (supra) the ankle bone (malleolus). SMOs are used to prevent the foot from excessively turning in or out or side to side while walking but still allow free ankle and toe movements. SMOs do not usually provide enough control if there is increased tone in the legs.

Shoe Inserts. Shoe inserts, the least restrictive type of bracing intervention, can be used for children who primarily need improved foot alignment but have good control of the knee and ankle. These fit inside the child's shoe, usually in place of the insole the shoe came with. These typically provide an increased arch support. They may be customized for your child's unique needs, but prefabricated versions are also commercially available.

Modifications to Braces. There are certain modifications that can be made to the brace to make it more effective for your child.

- The strength of the strut (the tall piece of plastic on an AFO that goes from the ankle to the calf) can be increased if your child has very high tone. The straps of the AFO can be strengthened and can be either stretch or non-stretch fabric, depending on the amount of control needed by your child.
- "Posting" can improve the foot position in standing. This involves modifying the bottom of the brace by adding extra material to build up the brace so that it helps maintain the foot flat on the floor in the improved alignment.
- Pads made of a variety of cushioned materials can be added to any brace, depending on the need. For example, toe pads can be added to help decrease muscle tone, or pads can be added to stabilize the heel and/or midfoot.

BRACING DURING SLEEP

According to your child's needs, he may wear his prescribed braces all or part of the day. Children do not typically wear their AFOs or DAFOs while they are sleeping. There are specialized orthoses made for nighttime use called resting night splints. These night splints may be used to supplement your child's daily stretching program, to maintain appropriate ankle alignment, and to prevent prolonged muscle shortening during sleep. These are usually a more comfortable version of your child's AFOs or DAFOs that are used during the day.

Occasionally, dynamic resting night splints may be recommended. These brace types are called dynamic because they can be gradually adjusted over time to help your child achieve improved range of motion. These splints are especially useful if your child has increased muscle tone and is going through a growth spurt.

If your child has increased tone in the hamstring muscles in the back of the thigh, knee immobilizers may be recommended. Knee immobilizers used for children with cerebral palsy are usually made of foam-padded fabric that wrap around your child's leg and are fastened with Velcro. The immobilizers include removable stays, usually made of aluminum, which are on each side of and behind the knee to prevent the knee from bending during sleep.

ORDERING BRACES

Orthoses are typically custom made out of high temperature plastics. A cast of your child's foot or ankle is made and then braces are customized from this cast. Although the initial casting is often completed by your physical therapist, the braces are usually fabricated by an orthotist, a specialist in constructing customized braces. It is important that you and your child work closely with both the orthotist and physical therapist to ensure proper fit and functioning of the braces.

Before actually ordering braces for your child, it will be helpful for you to sit down and make a list of things you think the braces should help your child accomplish. You and your therapist should discuss your child's skills and be mindful that bracing should not take away any of his function. You should then review all of these considerations with your therapist and orthotist to make sure that all of your child's needs are considered. Don't hesitate to ask questions. Everyone involved wants your child to get the correct fit and function from the braces. No one involved wants extra visits, revisions, or re-castings for your child. Revisions may be necessary, but some of these can often be avoided by careful planning and problem solving before your child's braces are ordered.

Parent education and active participation in any chosen intervention is crucial to the treatment and ultimate outcome for children with cerebral palsy. Asking questions is not only encouraged, it is vital. The following are common questions that occur in discussions between parents and their health care team about additional interventions for children with cerebral palsy.

Conclusion

Using the information provided in this chapter as a jumping off point, I hope that you will begin your own research to investigate which interventions might be best for you and your child. I hope you will remember to ask many questions and gather information from a variety of sources. Your doctor and other members of your professional team will be able to provide you more information about the interventions included in this chapter, as well as about other treatment options for your own child. I hope that this chapter has better prepared you to embark on your own unique journey with your child with cerebral palsy.

Frequently Asked Questions

Q. *"Are the interventions discussed covered by insurance?"*
A. Usually all of the interventions are covered by health insurance except shoe orthotics (even with a prescription for the orthotics). These shoe inserts are usually reasonably priced, however, so they can still be a viable treatment option.

Q. *"What are possible side effects of Baclofen? Do they differ depending on whether the medication is taken orally or received via the pump?"*
A. If the medicine is taken orally, often a much larger dose has to be taken to see the therapeutic effect of decreased spasticity. Side effects are more common with oral administration because of this. Side effects from oral Baclofen include increased drowsiness, reflux, and constipation.

With use of a pump, Baclofen withdrawal can occur if the medication is stopped or significantly reduced over a short period of time. This can cause increased muscle tone, profound sweating, skin itching "crawling" sensations without a rash, agitation, increased heart and breathing rate, fever, and seizures. Baclofen withdrawal can quickly become an emergency situation, and this is why consistent medical supervision and routine follow-up care are so crucial.

Overdose of Baclofen, although not very common, can cause drowsiness, decreased muscle tone, sleepiness, irregular breathing and apnea, and a decreased heart rate and rhythm.

Q. *"With ITB, how often do the pumps or catheters fail? What complications or mechanical problems do we have to watch out for?"*
A. Some complications that can occur after pump placement include infection at the pump, catheter, or incision site. There can also be drug-related problems of either overdose or withdrawal. There is an increased risk for seizures, constipation, and a cerebrospinal fluid leak, and a fluid pocket can form around the pump. Mechanically, the catheter may kink or disconnect, and a blockage or perforation may develop at the level of the catheter. The pump can also simply malfunction or dislodge. None of these complications are common now that the pump has been successfully used with children for several years.

Q. *"Can children with ITB still lie down and play on their stomachs? What if they get bumped at the pump site?"*
A. Four to six weeks after pump implantation, your child can play on his stomach without any risk to his pump. Minor bumps at the pump site typically are not harmful in any way to your child.

Q. *How is "how much" determined for each child to ensure the safety of botulinum toxin injections?*
A. The physician administering the botulinum toxin injections to your child will calculate the safe total dosage based on your child's body weight, location and size of muscle, and degree of spasticity.

Q. *"Can my child's spasticity come back after Selective Dorsal Rhizotomy?"*
A. In children diagnosed with spastic diplegia, return of spasticity after the surgery is rare. A few children with spastic quadriplegia have experienced a return of spasticity.

Q. *"Will my child need braces after the SDR surgery?"*
A. Most children need to use an ankle brace after surgery to properly align the foot during weight bearing activities, especially because of the temporary weakness in the leg muscles that often occurs after surgery. Your child's current braces may be modified for use after surgery, or your child may need to be fitted for new braces after the surgery. After the extensive rehabilitation period, your child may no longer require bracing to maintain appropriate foot and leg alignment during daily activities.

Q. *"My child has not been able to straighten his legs for some time. Will this SDR procedure help him finally get his legs straight?"*
A. This surgery will remove the underlying cause of your child's reduced range of motion (the spasticity) but it cannot affect a fixed and permanently shortened muscle/tendon unit (contracture). Your child might need serial casting or a surgical intervention to correct a more severe contracture that doesn't respond to an aggressive positioning and stretching program. Some neurosurgeons opt to have an orthopedic surgeon address these fixed contractures during the same operating time that the child is receiving the SDR, but this is not as common as having two separate procedures. Remember that SDR usually prevents any further orthopedic interventions, but it cannot undo an already formed contracture.

Q. *"Are there any precautions for serial casting?"*
A. Immediate cast removal is required if your child has muscle spasms, signs of a friction or pressure sore, evidence suggesting an allergic reaction to the casting materials, swelling or any other signs of constriction of your child's circulation, or if he refuses to bear weight on the cast foot.

Q. *"How often should my child wear the braces?"*
A. Initially, your child will probably wear his braces one hour on/one hour off, but this will usually be increased daily as tolerated by your child. Ultimately, the amount of time the braces are worn each day depends on the reason your child is wearing them.

An older child who wears his braces to improve function in walking will probably wear his braces most of his waking hours. For a younger child who is learning to crawl, sit, and kneel, the braces will likely interfere with these skills during floor playtime. For those younger children who primarily crawl, but also are beginning to stand and walk, it may be necessary to remove and replace the braces during the day to allow good floor mobility but to also encourage the child's new standing and walking skills.

For children who wear braces most of the day to maintain muscle length or functional skills, it is important to remember that they should have some time out of braces each day to allow the opportunity for muscle strengthening and freedom of movement, as overuse of braces may result in weakness, especially of the calf muscles.

The brace-wearing schedule is different for each child, depending upon his needs, and is something you should definitely discuss with your child's therapist.

Q. *"How will I know if the braces fit properly?"*
A. Daily skin checks are important to determine if the brace is putting abnormal pressure on your child's foot. An area of pressure can quickly turn into a blister and then a pressure sore if not found in the early stages. Any redness of the skin should go away within 15 minutes. If it remains longer, your child's braces need some adjustment to prevent further abnormal pressure. Your therapist will discuss this with you and give you further information about warning signs of skin breakdown.

Q. *"What kind of shoes should I get for my child to wear with his braces and how big should they be?*
A. Your child's braces are designed to provide him with maximum foot support so the shoes he wears is not the primary concern. However, it is important that the brace does not slip out of the shoe when your child is walking, and that the sole of the shoe is not slippery. The shoes are usually about one size larger than your child would wear without braces. The easiest way to find appropriate shoes for your child is to take the brace, without the foot in the brace, and slip it into various shoes until you find one that seems to fit well. Then have your child put the braces on and try the selected shoes.

Avoid heavy shoes, as they may overly tire your child's lower leg muscles when they are worn for long periods of time. Avoid shoes that are too long or too large because your child's balance and stability will be affected. Many children and families find lightweight sneakers or sport shoes to be the most comfortable and functional footwear to be worn over the braces.

Q. *"How will wearing ankle/foot braces affect my child's hip and knee position during standing and walking?*
A. It is an accepted fact that control of the foot may produce more control of the hip and knee. An easy way to understand this concept is to think of your child's leg as a chain with each link interconnected and the foot the primary link. If the primary link of the chain (the foot) is corrected into the appropriate alignment, it will positively affect the other connected links (hip and knee).

Q. *"Are there any negative effects of bracing?"*
A. It is possible that bracing may cause muscle weakness, especially in the muscles of the lower legs. This can happen in brace styles that prevent or limit movement at a

joint. The muscles that control the movement that is limited or prevented are at risk for increased weakness. Braces which result in an improved standing and walking pattern may also interfere with higher level gross motor activities such as running, hopping, and skipping. Because of these two concerns, professionals must ensure that the prescribed braces do not provide more assistance than a specific child needs.

If you believe that your child has lost muscle strength or functional skills as the result of his braces, discuss this with your physical therapist so that appropriate adjustments may be made to the braces and/or wearing schedule.

Q. *"Will my child ever outgrow his need for bracing?"*
A. Both you and your professional team must closely monitor the need for your child to continue with braces. If your child's muscle length becomes stable, as sometimes happens following growth, or if his muscle control improves, there may no longer be a need for braces. In other cases, additional interventions such as medication or surgery may improve strength, joint alignment, or function, resulting in a situation in which bracing is no longer recommended.

References

Albright, A.L. Intrathecal baclofen in cerebral palsy movement disorders. *Journal of Child Neurology,* 11(suppl 1):S29-S35, 1996.

Albright, A.L., Gilmartin, R., Swift, D., Krach, L.E., Ivanhoe, C.B., McLaughlin, J.F. Long-term intrathecal baclofen therapy for severe spasticity of cerebral origin. *Journal of Neurosurgery,* 98:291-295, 2003.

Albright, A.L., Meythaler, J.M., Ivanhoe, C.B. Intrathecal baclofen therapy for spasticity of cerebral origin: patient selection guidelines. Provided through an educational grant from Medtronic, Inc., 1997.

Baker, L.L., Wederich, C.L., McNeal, D.R., Newsam, C., Waters, R.L. *Neuro Muscular Electrical Stimulation: A Practical Guide,* 4th ed. Downey, CA: Rancho Los Amigos Research and Education Institute.

Barry, M.J., Albright, L.A., Shultz, B.L. Intrathecal baclofen therapy and the role of the physical therapist. *Pediatric Physical Therapy,* 12(2):77-86, 2000.

Buckon, C.E., Thomas, S.S., Piatt, J.H., Jr., Aiona, M.D., Sussman, M.D. Selective dorsal rhizotomy versus orthopedic surgery: A multidimensional assessment of outcome efficacy. *Archives of Physical Medicine Rehabilitation,* 85(3):457-485(3):457-465, 2004 Mar.

Buckon, C.E., Thomas, S.S., Harris, G.E., Piatt, J.H., Jr., Aiona, M.D., Sussman, M.D. Objective measurement of muscle strength in children with spastic diplegia after selective dorsal rhizotomy. *Archives of Physical Medicine Rehabilitation,* 83(4):454-460, 2002 Apr.

Campbell, S. (Ed.), Palisano, R.J., Vander Linden, D.W. *Physical Therapy for Children.* Philadelphia: W.B. Saunder, 1995.

Carmick, J. Guidelines for the clinical application of neuromuscular electrical stimulation for children with cerebral palsy. *Pediatric Physical Therapy,* 9:128-136, 1997.

Carmick, J. Managing equines in children with cerebral palsy: Electrical stimulation to strengthen the triceps surae muscle. *Developmental Medicine Child Neurology,* 37(11):965-975, 1995 Nov.

Carmick, J. Clinical use of neuromuscular electrical stimulation for children with cerebral palsy, part 1: lower extremity. *Physical Therapy,* 73(8):505-513, 1993 Aug.

Cusick, B. *Serial Casting to Restore Soft-tissue Extendability in the Ankle and Foot.* Placerville, CO: Progressive GaitWays, LLC, 2000.

Diener, C.E. Dynamic splinting of the lower extremity. Twelfth Annual School-Based OT/PT Institute, 2004.

Gaebler-Spira D., Revivo, G. The use of botulinum toxin in pediatric disorders. *Physical Medicine Rehabilitation Clinic of North America,* 14(4):703-725, 2003 Nov.

Gerszten, P.C., Albright, A.L., Johnstone, G.F. Intrathecal baclofen infusion and subsequent orthopedic surgery in patients with spastic cerebral palsy. *Journal of Neurosurgery,* 88:1009-1013, 1998.

Giorgetti, M.M. Serial and inhibitory casting: implications for acute care physical therapy management. *Neurology Report,* 17:18-21, 1993.

Gooch, J.L., Oberg, W.A., Grams, B., Ward, L.A., Walker, M.L. Care provider assessment of intrathecal baclofen in children. *Developmental Medicine and Child Neurology,* 46(8):548-552, 2004 Aug.

Gormley, M.E., Jr, Krach, L.E., Piccini, L. Spasticity management in the child with spastic quadriplegia. *European Journal of Neurology,* 8 Suppl 5:127-135, 2001 Nov.

Hagglund, G., Andersson, S., Duppe, H., Pedertsen, H.L., Nordmark, E., Westbom, L. Prevention of severe contractures might replace multilevel surgery in cerebral palsy: Results of a population-based health care programme and new techniques to reduce spasticity. *Journal of Pediatric Orthopedics,* 14(4):268-272, 2005 Jul.

Kinnett, D. Botulinum toxin A injections in children: Technique and dosing issues. *American Journal of Physical Medicine Rehabilitation,* 83(10 Suppl): S59-S64, 2004 Oct.

Mittal, S., Farmer, J.P., Al-Atassi, B., Montpetit, K., Gervais, N., Poulin, C., Benaroch, T.E., Cantin, MA. Functional performance following selective posterior rhizotomy: Long-term results determined using a validated evaluative measure. *Journal of Neurosurgery,* 97(3):510-518, 2002 Sep.

Plassat, R., Perrouin Verbe, B., Menei, P., Menegalli, D., Mathe, J.F., Richard, I. Treatment of spasticity with intrathecal Baclofen administration: long-term follow-up, review of 40 patients. *Spinal Cord,* 42(12):686-693, 2004 Dec.

Robinson, A.J., Snyder-Macklin, L. *Clinical Electrophysiology, Electrotherapy and Electrophysiologic Testing,* 2nd Ed. Baltimore: Williams & Wilkins, 1995.

Russman, B.S., Ashwal, S. Evaluation of the child with cerebral palsy. *Seminars in Pediatric Neurology,* 11(1):47-57, 2004.

Sgouros S., Seri S. The effect of intrathecal baclofen on muscle co-contraction in children with spasticity of cerebral origin. *Pediatric Neurosurgery,* 37(5):225-230, 2002 Nov.

Stackhouse, S.K., Binder-Macleod, S.A., Lee, S.C. Voluntary muscle activation, contractile properties, and fatigability in children with and without cerebral palsy. *Muscle Nerve,* 31(5):594-601, 2005 May.

Steinbok, P., Hicdonmez, T., Sawatzky, B., Beauchamp, R., Wickenheiser, D. Spinal deformities after selective dorsal rhizotomy for spastic cerebral palsy. *Journal of Neurosurgery,* 102(4 Suppl):363-373, 2005 May.

Tecklin, J.S. *Pediatric Physical Therapy,* 2nd Ed. Philadelphia: J.B. Lippincott, 1994.

Van Schie, P.E., Vermeulen, F.J., van Ouwerkerk, W.J., Dwakkel, G., Becher, J.G. Selective dorsal rhizotomy in cerebral palsy to improve functional abilities: Evaluation of criteria for selection. *Child's Nervous System,* 21(6):451-457, 2005 Jun.

Wong, A.M., Pei, Y.C., Lui, T.N., Chen, C.L., Wang, C.M., Chung, Cy. Comparison between botulinum toxin type A injections and selective posterior rhizotomy in improving gait performance in children with cerebral palsy. *Journal of Neurosurgery,* 102(4 Suppl):385-389, 2005 May.

Appendix

Pediatric Therapy Equipment

The following is a list of equipment that is mentioned or illustrated in this book. The items depicted in the photos were not specifically selected but shown because the child in the photo used them. With a few exceptions, the equipment is not needed to do the activities and exercises recommended, but parents may find it useful. Most of the equipment is manufactured by a variety of companies and available through pediatric equipment catalogs or online. Some of the items, including the large balls and Boppy pillows, are also available in retail stores that carry baby or sporting goods items. The last two items are not commercially available, but may be constructed following the given dimensions.

- Boppy Pillow (photo 6.14, page 65)
- Large Therapy Balls (photo 6.4, page 62)
- Therapy Wedge (photo 6.6, page 62)
- Therapy Rolls
- Adjustable Benches
- Adjustable Floor Table (photo 10.9a, page 102)
- Net Swing (photo 6.10, page 63)
- Scooter Board (photo 12.7, page 133)
- Immobilizers, for arms and legs
- Prone Stander (one model is shown in photo 6.14, page 65)
- Gait Trainer (one model is shown in photo 14.9, page 164)

- Forward Walker (one model is shown in photo 14.4, page 162)
- Reverse Walkers (one model is shown in photo 14.5, page 162)
- Forearm Crutches
- Adapted tricycle (photo 16.10a, page 205)
- Suction bars (photos 12.14a, b, c, page 137)
- Divider for gait training commercially available or made with 2 x 4 board placed on 2" edge and secured in place at both ends (photo 15.19a, page 196)
- Walking Ladder commercially available. May be used instead of ladder box, below
- Ladder box - the wooden box measures 12" L x 12" W x 7" H with 46" long extensions to increase stability and 22" H ladder extending off one side. Ladder rungs are 4½" apart. (Ladder box is shown in photo 12.17a and b, page 140)
- Standing (lean-to) board – 14" W with length adjusted for child, distance feet to middle chest (nipple line). Cut-out section at bottom accommodates feet. Board is padded with foam and covered with vinyl. (Standing board is illustrated in photo 12.12, page 136)

This list represents a mere fraction of the special-needs equipment available. Many of the items are designed for very specific use. Before purchasing equipment, parents are urged to discuss it thoroughly with their child's therapist. He or she will make sure that a piece of equipment is appropriate for your child. Good equipment should either help you take care of your child or foster his skill development.

General Equipment and Supplies

The following is a list of the supplies used with activities or exercises recommended in this book:

- Play table with a rim. The one shown in photos 15.1a and b (page 184) comes with 18.5" legs. A 24" leg kit is available to increase its height.
- Grab bars (photos 12.21a and b, page 142)
- Banister (photo 12.20, page 142)
- Bed tray (photos 10.3 and 10.9b, pages 98, 102)
- Wall bar (photo 12.21a, page 142)
- Storage crates of various sizes (photo 10.6, page 99)
- Laundry basket (photo 10.13, page 103)
- Notebook binder – substituting for therapy wedge (photo 11.2, page 121)
- Beanbags and box or bucket (photos 13.7 snf 15.18, pages 149, 194)
- Sand bags, three to six pounds, made by sewing up the legs of old jeans and filling them with sand (photo 10.7, page 100)
- Wrist and ankle weights, three to seven pounds; best with Velcro closure (photos 6.13 and 10.8a, b, pages 65, 101)
- Hand weights, a quarter pound or half pound (photo 13.2, page 148)

- Homemade hand weights – place a quarter or half a pound of dried beans in a tube sock. Shake beans to center and tie sock into knots at both ends.
- Balls—small balls, playground ball, larger lightweight balls, beach ball
- Rings, as used for a ring toss game or for diving (photo 12.6, page 133)
- Hoop (photos 14.18a and b; 15.21, pages 169, 197)
- Sticks, a broomstick cut in half or into three or four pieces (photos 13.13 and 14.11, pages 151, 165)
- Foam squares the size of seat cushions (photo 15.14, page 192)
- Balloons of various sizes
- Shaving cream and foam shapes

Therapy Equipment Suppliers

Here is a small sample of companies that sell pediatric therapy equipment that may be of use to parents of children with cerebral palsy. There are many other good sources; ask your physical therapist what companies he or she recommends.

Abilitations
P.O. Box 922668
Norcross, GA 30010
800-850-8602
www.abilitations.com

Achievement Products
P. O. Box 9033
Canton, OH 44711
800-766-4303
www.specialkidszone.com

Danmar Products, Inc.
221 Jackson Industrial Drive
Ann Arbor, MI 48103
800-783-1998
danmarpro@aol.com

Equipment Shop
P.O. Box 33
Bedford, MA 01730
800-525-7681
www.equipmentshop.com

Flaghouse
Rehab Resources
601 Flaghouse Dr.
Hasbrouck Heights, NJ 07604
800-793-7900
www.FlagHouse.com

Kaye Products
535 Dimmocks Mill Road
Hillsborough, NC 27278
919-732-6444
www.kayeproducts.com

Nilo
4011 Avenida De La Plata, #302
Oceanside, CA 92056
800-872-6456
www.nilotoys.com
(Supplier of play table with rim)

Rifton Equipment
359 Gibson Hill Road
Chester, NY 10918
800-777-4244
www.rifton.com

Sammons Preston Rolyan Pediatrics
An AbilityOne Company
P.O. Box 5071
Bolingbrook, IL 60440
800-323-5547
www.sammonsprestonrolyan.com

Organizations Providing Recreational Opportunities

Little League Challenger Division
Little League Baseball Headquarters
P.O. Box 3485
Williamsport, PA 17701
www.littleleague.org/divisions/challenger.asp

National Sports Center for the Disabled
P.O. Box 1290
Winter Park, CO 80482
970-726-1540
www.nscd.org

North American Riding for the Handicapped Association (NRHA)
P.O. Box 33150
Denver, CO
800-369-7433
NARHA@NARHA.org

Special Olympics
1133 19th Street, NW
Washington, DC 20036
202-628-3630
www.specialolympics.org

U.S. Youth Soccer TOPSoccer
www.youthsoccer.org/programs/topsoccer
1-800-4SOCCER
Chairman Susanne Conlons, conlons@mindspring.com

Wheelchair Sports USA
1668 320th Way
Earlham, IA 50072
515 833-2450
www.wsusa.org

References

Ahl Ekstrom, L. et al. Functional therapy for children with cerebral palsy: An ecological approach. *Developmental Medicine and Child Neurology* 2005;47:613-619.

Bandy, W.D. et al. The effect of static stretch and dynamic range of motion training on the flexibility of the hamstring muscles. *Journal of Orthopaedic and Sports Physical Therapy* 1998;27:295-300.

Bandy, W.D. et al. The effect of time and frequency of static stretching on flexibility of hamstring muscles. *Physical Therapy* 1997;77:1090-1096.

Bleck, E.E. The locomotor prognosis in cerebral palsy. *Developmental Medicine and Child Neurology* 1975;17:18-25.

Bobath, K. *The Neurophysiological Basis for the Treatment of Cerebral Palsy.* Clinics in Developmental Medicine, No. 75. London: William Heinemann Medical Books, 1980.

Cotton E. *Conductive Education and Cerebral Palsy.* London: The Spastic Society, 1974.

Day, J.A. et al. Locomotor training with partial body weight support on a treadmill in a nonambulatory child with spastic tetraplegic cerebral palsy: A case report. *Pediatric Physical Therapy* 2004;16:106-113.

Dodd, K.J., Graham, H.K.. A randomized clinical trial of strength training in young people with cerebral palsy. *Developmental Medicine and Child Neurology* 2003;45:652-657.

Eagleton, M. et al. The effects of strength training on gait in adolescents with cerebral palsy. *Pediatric Physical Therapy* 2004;1622-30.

Engsberg, J.R. et al. Changes in hip spasticity and strength following selective dorsal rhizotomy and physical therapy for spastic cerebral palsy. *Developmental Medicine and Child Neurology* 2002;44:220-226.

Feland, J.B. et al. The effect of duration of stretching of the hamstring muscle group for increasing range of motion in people aged 65 years or older. *Physical Therapy* 2001;81:1111-1117.

Finnie, N.R. *Handling the Young Child with Cerebral Palsy at Home.* Third edition. Edinburgh: Butterworth-Heinemann, 1997.

Fowler, E.G. et al. The effect of quadriceps femoris muscle strengthening exercises on spasticity in children with cerebral palsy. *Physical Therapy* 2001;81:1215-1223.

Fragala-Pinkham, M.A. et al. A fitness program for children with disabilities. *Physical Therapy* 2005;85:1182-1200.

Folio, M.R., Fewell, R.R. *Peabody Developmental Motor Scales.* Second edition. Austin, TX: PRO-ED, 2000.

Geralis, E. *Children with Cerebral Palsy: A Parent's Guide.* Second edition. Bethesda, MD: Woodbine House, 1998.

Jaeger, L. and Gertz, J. *Home Program Instruction Sheets for Infants and Children.* San Antonio: Therapy Skill Builders, 1997.

Ketelaar, M et al. Effect of functional therapy program on motor abilities of children with cerebral palsy. *Physical Therapy* 2001;81:1534-45

Lespargot, A. et al. Stretching the triceps surae muscle after 40 degrees C warming in patients with cerebral palsy. *Revue de Chirugie Orthopedique Reparatrice de L'Appareil Moteur* 2000,86:712-7.

McBurney, H. et al. A qualitative analysis of the benefits of strength training for young people with cerebral palsy. *Developmental Medicine and Child Neurology* 2003;45:658-663.

Nash, J. et al. Reducing spasticity to control muscle contracture of children with cerebral palsy. *Developmental Medicine and Child Neurology* 1989,31:471-480.

O'Dwyer, N.J., Neilson, P.D., Nash, J. Mechanisms of muscle growth related to muscle contracture in cerebral palsy. *Developmental Medicine and Child Neurology* 1989,31:543-552.

Palisano, R.J. et al. Validation of a model of gross motor function for children with cerebral palsy. *Physical Therapy* 2000;80:974-985.

Pax Lowes, L. et al. Muscle force and range of motion as predictors of standing balance in children with cerebral palsy. *Physical & Occupational Therapy in Pediatrics* 2004;24:57-77.

Rosenbaum et al. Prognosis for gross motor function in cerebral palsy: Creation of motor developmental curves. *Journal of the American Medical Association* 2002;288:1357-1363.

Ross, S.A., Engsberg, J.R. Relation between spasticity and strength in individuals with spastic diplegic cerebral palsy. *Developmental Medicine and Child Neurology* 2002;44:148-157.

Russel, D.J. et al. *Gross Motor Function Measure.* Cambridge: Gross Motor Measures Group, 1990.

Russel D.J. et al. *Gross Motor Function Measure: A Measure of Gross Motor Function in Cerebral Palsy.* (GMFM-66 and GMFM-88) Cambridge, 2002.

Shumway-Cook, A., Woollacott, M.H. *Motor Control: Theory and Practical Application.* Second edition. Baltimore: Lippincott Williams & Wilkins, 2001.

Stuberg, W.A. et al. Effects of manual stretching on hamstring flexibility in children with cerebral palsy. Unpublished, 2005.

Thorpe, D.E., Valvano, J. The effects of knowledge of performance and cognitive strategies on motor skill learning in children with cerebral palsy. *Pediatric Physical Therapy* 2002; 14:2-15.

Westcott, S.L., Burtner, P. Postural control in children: Implications for pediatric practice. *Physical & Occupational Therapy in Pediatrics* 2004;24:5-55.

Wood, E.P., Rosenbaum, P.L. The Gross Motor Function Classification System for Cerebral Palsy: A study of reliability and stability over time. *Developmental Medicine and Child Neurology* 2000;42:292-296.

Index

Intrathecal baclofen (ITB), 210–11, 217, 218
Joint contracture, 43–44, 214
Joint problems, 42–44
Joint stabilization, 32–33
Joint subluxation/dislocation, 43
Kinetic chain exercises, 31–32
Kneeling, 106, 125, 126, 150–52, 154
Knee walking, 151
Ladder, 140
Leg exercises, 132–34, 136–38
Leg movements, stimulating, 131
Leg stretching, 49–52, 56
Martial arts, 207
Massed practice, 29
Medical intervention, 209–12
Medications, 210
Motivation, 60
Motor control/coordination, lack of, 21–22
Motor development, obstacles to, 17–23
Motor learning, principles, 26–29
Motor skills, learning, 25–40. *See also* Gross motor
    development
  controlled weight shifts and, 31
  dissociating and, 33
  joint stabilization and, 32–33
  kinetic chain exercises and, 31–32
  massed practice and, 29
  neural plasticity and, 25
  physical therapy treatments and, 29–35
  principles of, 26–29
  self-stabilization and, 34–35
  stabilization techniques and, 33–34
  teaching functional skills and, 35
  weight bearing and, 30–31
Movement patterns, 19
Muscle/joint flexibility, 41–56
  daily stretching and, 42, 43, 44–45
  joint contracture and, 43
  joint subluxation/dislocation and, 43
  problems and, 41–42
  stretching exercises and, 45–52
Muscle tone, 17–18. *See also* Spasticity
Muscles, 17–22
  balance and, 145
  control of, 21, 22
  extensor, 8
  flaccid, 17

flexor, 7
floor sitting and, 100
leg exercises and, 132, 133, 134
length of, 41–45
lower extremity bracing and, 214
problems with, 41-42
sitting and, 108, 109
strength exercises and, 201–03
weakness of, 22
Neural plasticity, 25
Neurodevelopment Treatment (NDT), 30. *See also*
    Bobath, Bertha
Neuromuscular electrical stimulation (NMES), 213–14
Oral medications, 210
Orthopedic surgery, 211, 213, 214
Orthoses. *See* Braces
Palisano, Robert, 11
Parachute response, 88, 89, 90–92
Passive range of motion (PROM), 43
Pediatric therapy equipment, 221–24
Peto ladder, 140
Physical therapist
  back-lying and, 68, 71, 72
  bench sitting and, 109
  "big arm" exercises and, 80
  braces and, 214, 216
  crawling and, 117
  developmental delay and, 1
  gross motor development and, 10
  gross motor skills and, 79
  head control and, 57, 66
  joint stabilization and, 33
  motor learning and, 26
  neuromuscular electrical stimulation (NMES)
    and, 213
  self-stabilization and, 34–35
  serial casting and, 213
  sitting and, 95
  standing balance and, 153
  stretching exercises and, 45, 46, 47, 48, 49, 54
  tummy time exercises and, 76–78
  walkers and, 161–64
  weight bearing and, 30–31, 88–89
  weight shifts and, 31
Physical therapy, 29-35, 118, 153, 212
Physiological flexion, 67
Prone position. *See* Stomach-lying

About the author:

Sieglinde Martin, M.S., P.T., is a physical therapist with more than thirty years of clinical experience working with children with cerebral palsy and their families. Ms. Martin earned her degree in physical therapy from the University of Cologne, Germany, and her Master's of Science degree at Ohio State University in Columbus, Ohio. Currently she works part-time at Children's Close To Home Health Care Center in Dublin, Ohio. She is also the author of *Pediatric Balance Program* (Therapy Skill Builders, 1998).